Real Medicine, Unreal Stories

Lessons and Insights from Clinical Practice

Volume 1

Arthur Lazarus, MD, MBA

ISBN: 978-1-965469-80-4

Also by Arthur Lazarus

Neuroleptic Malignant Syndrome and Related Conditions (co-author)

Controversies in Managed Mental Health Care

Career Pathways in Psychiatry: Transition in Changing Times

MD/MBA: Physicians on the New Frontier of Medical Management

Every Story Counts: Exploring Contemporary Practice Through Narrative Medicine

Medicine on Fire: A Narrative Travelogue

Narrative Medicine: The Fifth Vital Sign

Narrative Medicine: Harnessing the Power of Storytelling through Essays

Story Treasures: Medical Essays and Insights in the Narrative Tradition

21st Century Schizoid Health Care: Essays and Reflections to Keep You Sane on Your Medical Travels

Narrative Rx: A Quick Guide to Narrative Medicine for Students, Residents, and Attendings

Narrative Medicine: New and Selected Essays

Author's Note

This book was inspired by real people and events. However, the stories, characters, and outcomes have been significantly altered or combined, and should therefore be considered fictional.

All stories were written in early 2025. Illustrations were created by ChatGPT and are subject to limitations inherent in AI-generated content.

This book contains descriptions of suicide and suicidal ideation. If you or someone you know is struggling or in crisis, help is available at *the National Suicide Prevention Lifeline*. Call or text 988 or chat at 988lifeline.org.

Nothing in this book should be used as a substitute for medical advice from a doctor or other qualified healthcare professional.

Dedication

To John R. ("Jack") Benson, M.D. —

May his memory be a blessing, as it has been to me,
and may it continue to guide all who had the privilege of knowing him.

Table of Contents

"The lies that people tell in stories is what makes them so true."

— Majid Kazmi

Preface

People often describe medicine as both an art and a science, a delicate balance between knowledge and intuition, precision and human connection. Yet, for all its rigor and scientific advancements, the practice of medicine remains deeply entwined with story — narratives of patients and physicians, of healing and suffering, of discovery and loss. Real Medicine, Unreal Stories: Lessons and Insights from Clinical Practice is born from this intersection, weaving together fictionalized accounts inspired by real-world medical encounters to reveal deeper truths about the profession.

Fiction, paradoxically, has the power to illuminate reality in ways that raw facts and statistics cannot. Through fictional narrative, we can easily enter the minds of doctors facing impossible ethical dilemmas, patients grappling with diagnoses that redefine their lives, and healthcare systems straining under the weight of bureaucracy. The stories in this book are not mere entertainment (although I hope that purpose is served); they are invitations to reflect on the complexities, contradictions, and moral ambiguities inherent in modern medicine. The aim is to offer insight, compassion, and humor while shedding light on the challenging realities of medical practice.

Each piece explores a distinct facet of clinical medicine: the triumphs and failures, the moments of doubt and fortitude, and the conflicts between evidence-based care and human instincts. Some stories dissect the inner struggles of physicians—the burden of responsibility, the weight of a lost patient, the quiet victories that keep them going. Others highlight the evolving landscape of health care, from artificial intelligence to the ethical implications of cutting-edge treatments, from the depersonalization of medicine to the fragile trust between patient and doctor.

Though the characters and scenarios are fictional, the emotions they evoke are very real. They echo the lived experiences of countless doctors, nurses, residents, medical students, and patients contending with an imperfect system. We aim to challenge, provoke, and inspire these stories, reminding us that medicine is fundamentally a human endeavor.

For those who have lived these moments—who have faced the late-night decisions, the gut-wrenching diagnoses, and the ethical tightropes—I hope these stories resonate with your experiences, affirming the challenges you have endured and the tenacity that sustains you. This book shows the science and soul of medicine to those new to the field or outside of it.

Welcome to *Real Medicine, Unreal Stories*—where every story contains a lesson, and every lesson is a reflection of the path we travel in the pursuit of healing.

1. No Screen Time for Jake

A doctor explains how a digital drug is rewiring childhood.

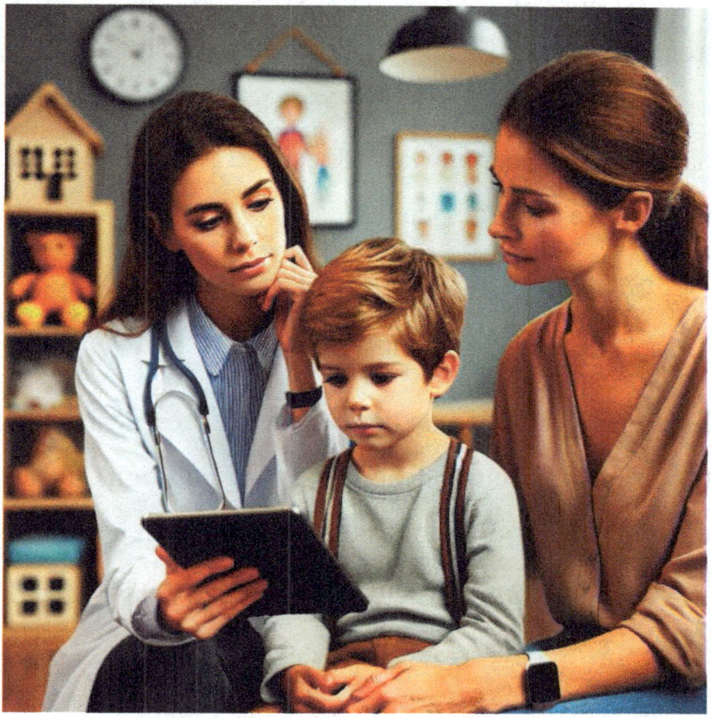

Dr. Samantha Ryan glanced at the clock. It was five minutes past four. She sighed, knowing the last patient of the day always came with an extra layer of exhaustion.

She knocked. "Come in," a voice called from the other side of the door.

A frazzled woman in her mid-30s—an established patient—was clutching the hand of her son, who couldn't have been older than six. He was glued to a tablet, his eyes wide, fingers rapidly tapping the screen.

"Dr. Ryan, I'm worried about Jake. He's had a bit of trouble sleeping lately, and he's been struggling in school." The woman, Laura, exhaled deeply, running a hand through her unwashed hair. "I was hoping you might have some advice."

Dr. Ryan motioned for them to sit. "Tell me more. Trouble sleeping? Difficulty focusing?"

Laura nodded. "He just doesn't seem...present. He used to be such a curious kid, always asking questions, always outside playing. But now, he's obsessed with his screen. If I take it away, he has meltdowns. Full-on screaming, tears, the works."

Dr. Ryan glanced at Jake, who hadn't looked up once. "Jake, can I see that for a second?" She asked gently.

Jake hesitated but handed over the tablet. The screen was a swirl of fast-moving animations, bright colors, and flashing ads.

"What is this?" she asked.

“It’s a game,” Jake mumbled, barely audible.

Dr. Ryan turned to Laura. “How much screen time does he get per day?”

Laura winced. “I try to keep it under three hours, but honestly, some days it’s more. He’s always asking for it, and when I say no, the tantrums are unbearable. It’s just...easier.”

Dr. Ryan leaned forward, her expression kind but firm. “Laura, what if I told you that screen time is likely the reason for Jake’s struggles? It's not just a distraction; it's fundamentally changing his brain.”

Laura frowned. “I mean, I’ve read about it a little, but...it’s everywhere. What am I supposed to do? Keep him in a bubble?”

Dr. Ryan smiled. “Not a bubble” But boundaries. Right now, Jake’s brain is adapting to a world of instant gratification. Every time he plays a game, watches a video, or gets a notification, his brain releases dopamine—the same chemical linked to addiction. The more he uses screens, the harder it is for him to enjoy anything else.”

Laura sighed. "That explains a lot. He used to love playing outside. Now, I can barely get him to go to the park."

"Exactly," Dr. Ryan nodded. "It's called a 'dopamine loop.' Apps and games are designed to keep him hooked. When the screen disappears, he experiences withdrawal, which leads to his meltdowns.

Laura gestured, questioning. "So, what do I do? Take it away completely? Won't he just find another way to get it? I feel like I'm constantly fighting him."

Dr. Ryan handed the tablet back to Jake, who snatched it eagerly. "It's not about punishment—it's about rewiring his brain. The goal is to bring back his ability to enjoy real life again."

"How?"

"Start small. First, create 'no-screen zones'—dinner, the car, bedtime. Then, introduce screen-free activities he loves. Maybe reading, building Legos, or playing outside. And most importantly, replace screen time with a connection. Play with him, take him on adventures, show him the world beyond this tiny screen."

Laura hesitated. "That sounds...hard."

Dr. Ryan was sympathetic. “It will be. At first. He’ll resist. But kids don’t crave screens—they crave engagement. Right now, his brain just doesn’t remember how to enjoy anything else.”

Laura looked at Jake, who was still staring at his tablet, completely oblivious. “And if I don’t?”

Dr. Ryan’s face grew serious. “The research isn’t just concerning—it’s alarming. Excessive screen time has been linked to increased anxiety, depression, attention issues, and even changes in brain development. Kids today are struggling with focus, empathy, and deep thinking. Their childhoods are disappearing.”

Laura swallowed hard. “I don’t want that for him.” Then a long pause. “The funny thing is...my dad—he’s always been a great fan of Pete Townshend and The Who—they were well before my time. Dad’s always quoting Townshend about how the kids are ‘alright.’ It’s a song, he tells me”.

“Well, I hate to disrupt your dad’s song and dance routine, but the kids are not alright. You’ve got to start today. Cut back the screen time. Make him bored again.

Boredom leads to creativity. Frustration leads to resilience. Let him rediscover childhood."

Laura took a deep breath. "Okay. We'll try."

Jake looked up for the first time. "Mom? Does that mean no screen time for me?"

Laura hesitated, then met Dr. Ryan's gaze. "That's exactly what it means."

For the first time all day, Dr. Ryan saw something change in Jake's eyes. Not frustration. Not sadness.

But curiosity.

And that was a start.

2. The Clash Between Science and Trust

A doctor balances skepticism, control, and belief in medical practice.

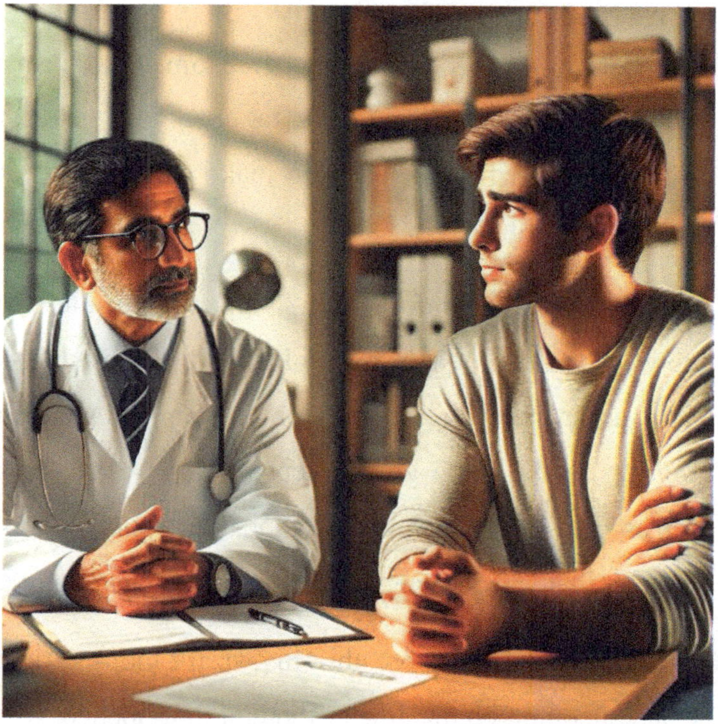

Dr. Amit Mehta sat back in his chair and folded his hands. He had seen that look before—the wary, crossed-arm stance of a patient who had already made up his mind. Spencer Frye, 32, had come in for what was supposed to be a routine physical, but the conversation had veered sharply into deep distrust.

“Look, doc, I get it. You have protocols, guidelines, or whatever you want to call them. But at the end of the day, shouldn’t I have the freedom to choose what’s best for my body?” Spencer asked.

“Absolutely, Spencer. You do have freedom. My job isn’t to force anything on you—it’s to give you the best possible information so you can make a decision that keeps you healthy.”

“Yeah, but whose information?” Spencer wanted to know. “The same people who told us sugar was safe—that smoking wasn’t that bad at one point? Are you referring to the same government that allowed events such as Tuskegee? Do you expect me to put blind trust in a system that’s been lying to people for decades?”

Dr. Mehta took a deep breath. This wasn’t the first time he had encountered this line of thought, but Spencer was clearly well-read — he wasn’t just parroting internet conspiracies.

“Spencer, I hear you. And you’re right—there have been dark chapters in medical history. The Tuskegee syphilis experiments that you refer to, Nazi medical atrocities, and even unethical corporate influence in science. Those were real, and they were horrific."

Spencer seemed momentarily surprised at the agreement. "Exactly! So why trust any of it?"

"Because science is not a monolith. It's not one person, one organization, or one government. It's a self-correcting process. Those tragedies happened because people in power abused science for their ends. But how do we even know they were unethical? Because scientific scrutiny exposed them. The same process that uncovered those abuses is the one that helps protect us today."

"But what about now? How do I know today's 'official science' isn't just another scam waiting to be exposed?"

"Good question. The key difference is transparency and oversight. Look at how medical guidelines are formed—studies go through peer review, research is replicated, and independent experts weigh in. And when mistakes happen, they get corrected. You mentioned the sugar industry influencing dietary guidelines decades ago. That was a problem, and now we have stronger disclosure rules and more rigorous studies to counter industry bias. Science learns from its failures."

Spencer rubbed his chin. "Still, government agencies control a lot of what gets funded, what gets approved. And we've seen a lot of politics messing with science lately."

Dr. Mehta nodded, referencing the changes in the administration Spencer had read about. "That's fair. There have been concerning moves—like restricting public input on policy changes at HHS or rolling back scientific oversight in environmental regulations. Those kinds of shifts can undermine trust. But again, what happens when bad policy suppresses good science? Scientists, doctors, and even patients push back. Just last week, researchers rallied in Washington to fight for transparency and funding for independent research."

"So, you're saying the system isn't perfect, but it's better than the alternative?"

"I'm saying medicine isn't about faith—it's about evidence. If you don't trust a government agency, look at the studies themselves. See how they're conducted, who funds them, and whether they've been replicated. Skepticism is healthy—it drives better science. But rejecting science entirely because of past abuses? That leaves you with nothing but guesswork."

"I just don't like feeling like I have no control."

Dr. Mehta moved closer. "You do have control. But control doesn't mean ignoring the best available knowledge—it means using it wisely. Think about seatbelts. The government mandates them, but you don't wear one because of a law. You wear one because, statistically, it saves your life. Medical science is the same way—it's not about control; it's about giving you the best shot at a long, healthy life."

Spencer looked introspectively at the pamphlet on health screenings, "Your 30s: Building a Foundation for Lifelong Health," that was on the table.

"Now is the time to establish habits that prevent chronic disease later in life," Dr. Mehta commented.

Spencer sat quietly for a moment, then picked up the pamphlet. "Alright, doc. I'll think about it."

Dr. Mehta smiled. That was all he could ask for.

3. All in Her Head

A doctor discusses how chronic pain sufferers are often mislabeled and delegitimized.

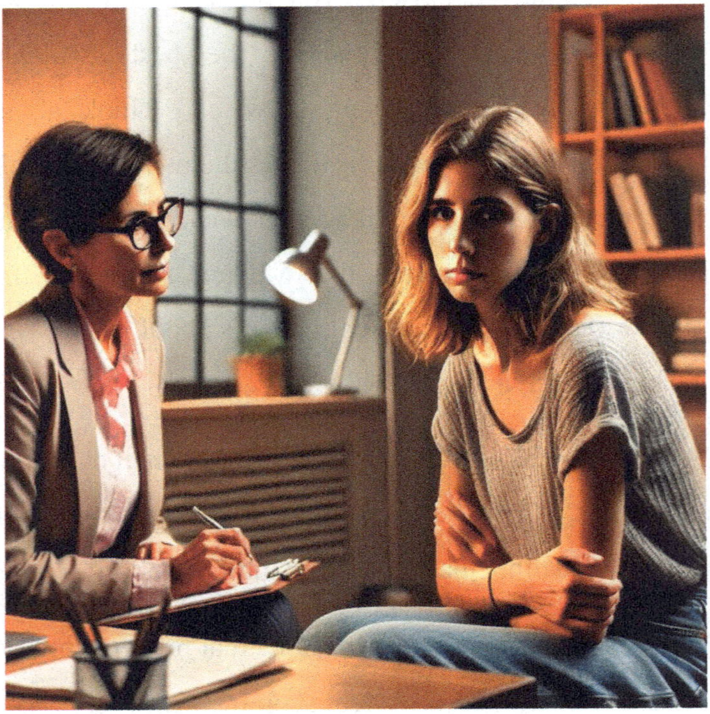

Dr. Rachel Feldman, a psychiatrist in her late 40s, sat across from a woman who appeared rigid, as if she were bracing herself for bad news. Sarah Lawson, 28, had been referred by her primary care physician—though "referred" was a generous term.

"He told me to see a psychiatrist," Sarah said flatly. "Because apparently, my pain isn't real. It's just my 'anxiety acting up.'"

Dr. Feldman stopped taking notes. "Tell me about your pain, Sarah."

A flicker of surprise crossed Sarah's face, but she quickly buried it. "I have fibromyalgia. At least, that's what one doctor finally called it after years of being told it was nothing." She let out a sharp laugh. "I saw my PCP last week because the pain has been unbearable, and do you know what he said? That maybe I just needed therapy. That women tend to 'somaticize stress' and that I should 'work through it emotionally.'"

"That must have been frustrating. What are your symptoms?"

Sarah reeled them off as if she were at a recital: pain…all over, fatigue, insomnia, concentration problems, stiffness, and headaches.

"You know what the worst part is?" Sarah asked. "If I were a man, he wouldn't have said that. If my boyfriend walked into his office complaining of pain, I bet he'd order labs and X-rays before he even finished his sentence."

Dr. Feldman had seen this pattern before. More often than men, the medical field dismissed women, especially those with chronic pain. Studies had shown that conditions like fibromyalgia were disproportionately diagnosed in women, yet the medical field still viewed them through a lens of skepticism.

"Sarah, you're not imagining this. What you're describing happens to many women. Pain, especially when it can't be neatly explained by a scan or a lab test, gets waved off as 'hysteria'—even now, in the 21st century. That term—hysteria—has been around since the ancient Greeks. Hippocrates believed that hysteria was a condition caused by a 'wandering womb,' where the uterus moved throughout the body, leading to various physical and psychological symptoms in women. Can you believe that?"

Sarah stared at Dr. Feldman, the tension in her shoulders softening just a little. "So, you actually believe me?"

"Of course, I do."

There was a beat of silence. Sarah looked down at her hands. “I don't even know why I'm here. I’m not crazy. I’m in pain.”

“And pain is exhausting. It grinds you down, wears away at you until there’s nothing left but frustration and despair. It’s no wonder that about half of people with fibromyalgia experience depression and anxiety.”

Sarah sighed. “Yeah… I feel like I’m drowning in it.”

“That doesn’t mean your pain isn’t real. It means your body is fighting on two fronts—physically and mentally. And that’s not because you’re weak; it’s because pain changes the brain. The longer it lasts, the more the nervous system rewires itself, making it harder to shut off.”

Sarah blinked, processing this. “So… Am I not just overreacting?”

“Not even close.”

For the first time, Sarah’s eyes welled with something apart from frustration. She gulped. “Then what do I do?”

“First, we address both the pain and the depression together. That doesn’t mean ignoring the pain in favor of mental health—because that's precisely what's been happening to you. It means treating both as real, because they are."

Sarah nodded slowly. "That makes sense."

"We'll talk about treatment options—medications, cognitive behavioral therapy, even pain management strategies that are backed by scientific research. And we'll make sure that the doctors you see next actually listen to you and take you seriously."

Sarah let out a breath she hadn't realized she was holding. "That would be a first."

Dr. Feldman smiled. "Then let's make it happen."

For the first time in years, Sarah felt something close to hope.

4. Uncharted Territory

A doctor is confronted with the dilemma of providing transgender treatment to minors.

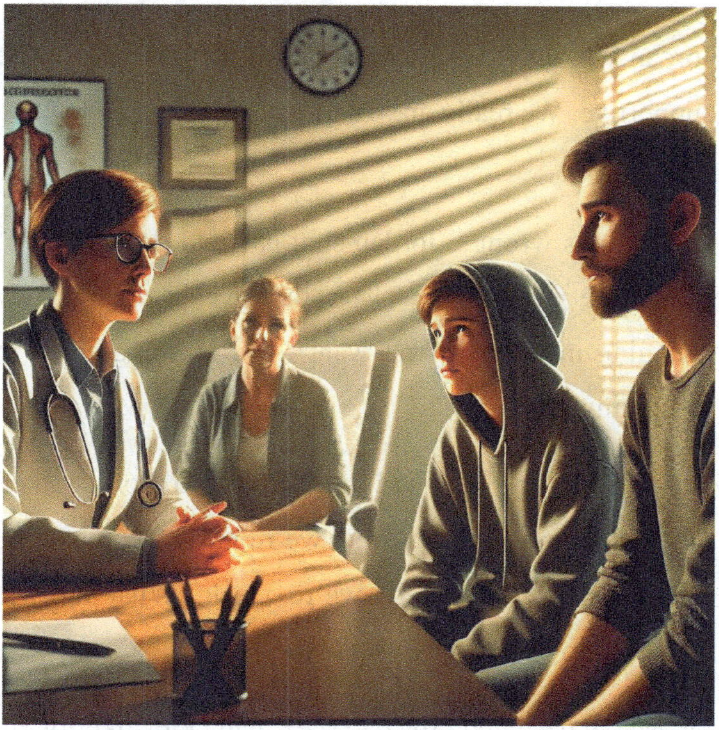

"I just...I don't know what else to do," Jordan's voice wavered, his fingers locked together so tightly his knuckles turned white. "I've known since I was little that something wasn't right. I'm supposed to be a girl."

Dr. Evelyn Marsh was unfazed, her hands folded on the desk between them. “Jordan, I hear you. And I know this isn't easy. But the law in our state prohibits me from prescribing puberty blockers or hormone therapy until you’re eighteen.”

Jordan’s mother, Lisa, chimed in. “We’re trying to be supportive. We really are. But this is...a lot. And the law is the law.”

“The law is wrong,” Jordan shot back. “I don’t want to wait three more years. That's three years of my body changing in ways I don't want—of becoming stuck in something I can't fix.”

His father, Mark, who had been silent until now, wanted to go on record. “Look, Doc, we’re not unsympathetic. But even if we agreed, we’re stuck. What are we supposed to do?”

Dr. Marsh hesitated. She had seen many kids like Jordan before, struggling against a system that often felt indifferent. “There are options,” she said carefully. “Social transition—changing pronouns, name, clothing Therapy with someone who understands gender dysphoria. But medical transition? Currently, it’s legally off the table.”

She gazed around the room before continuing. "The opposition to gender-affirming therapy comes largely from concerns over long-term effects, fears of regret, and the belief that minors lack the maturity to make such permanent decisions. Some argue that therapy should focus on helping individuals accept their birth sex rather than altering their bodies. They view medical transition as experimental, citing cases of detransition as proof of the need for greater caution.

She shifted slightly in her chair. "On the other side, medical professionals, including the American Academy of Pediatrics and the American Medical Association, recognize that gender dysphoria is real and that delaying treatment can lead to severe psychological distress. Gender-affirming care has been shown to reduce rates of depression and suicide among trans youth. For many, waiting until eighteen is not just difficult—it's devastating."

Jordan shook his head. "Explanations don't help. Everyone says I should just wait, but they don't understand how bad this feels. It's like being locked in a room where the walls are closing in, and no one will open the door."

Lisa reached out, hesitating before placing her hand over Jordan's. "We do get that you're hurting, honey. We're just scared, too. We hear all the political talk, and it's hard to know what's right."

Dr. Marsh added, "The unfortunate reality is that the issue has become more about politics than medicine. The consensus from medical professionals is clear—gender-affirming care can be life-saving. But in this state, lawmakers have decided otherwise."

Mark shifted in his chair. "And what about therapy? The kind that"— he hesitated, choosing his words —"helps kids work through their feelings, maybe find peace without medical intervention?"

Jordan's eyes widened. "You mean conversion therapy?" He turned to Dr. Marsh, alarmed. "That's illegal too, right?"

She nodded. "Yes. Bans on conversion therapy are in place to protect LGBTQ+ youth from harmful practices. The American Psychiatric Association repudiated conversion therapy years ago. But some providers—under the guise of counseling—offer what they call "exploratory therapy.' It's a gray area."

"I don't need therapy to convince me I'm wrong," Jordan muttered. "I need help."

Dr. Marsh shrugged her shoulders. "I wish I could do more. Some families in states with laws like this travel elsewhere for care, but I know that's not feasible for everyone."

Lisa looked at Mark, her expression conflicted. "What do we do? I don't want to lose our child."

Mark's voice was gruff. "We don't have all the answers. But we're not turning away from you, Jordan. We'll figure this out."

Jordan exhaled, looking between them. "You promise?"

Lisa squeezed his hand. "We promise."

Dr. Marsh nodded. "And in the meantime, we work with what we can. You have an ally in me, Jordan. Even if my hands are tied."

Jordan nodded, blinking back tears. The battle wasn't over, but for now, he wasn't alone.

5. The Battle Within

After losing a patient, a surgeon struggles with his identity and regains his confidence.

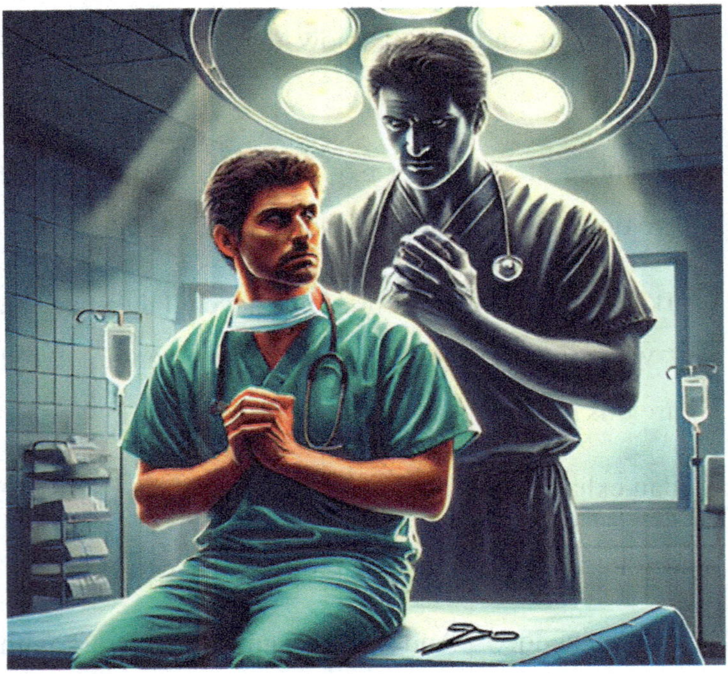

The hospital's surgical wing pulsed with quiet energy, a world in constant motion just beyond the break room's closed door. Inside, the dim light cast long shadows as Dr. Jonathan Meyers gazed down at his hands, which had unconsciously taken on a prayerful position.

His hands looked the same. But they weren't. And there was good reason for him to pray.

The door swung open, and Dr. Alan Pierce stepped inside, the scent of antiseptic clinging to his scrubs. "Jonathan, we need to talk."

"There's nothing to talk about." Jonathan's voice was hollow. "It's done. I made a mistake. Mr. Jameson is dead."

Pierce exhaled. "It was a rupture you couldn't have foreseen. You did everything you could."

Jonathan's laugh was bitter, barely a sound. "But I didn't, did I? I hesitated for a second. I second-guessed myself. If I had moved faster, if I had trusted—"

"If, if, if." Pierce stepped closer. "You know this game gets you nowhere."

Jonathan closed his eyes. "It gets me to the only place I deserve to be: out of the OR. Permanently."

Pierce's jaw tightened. "You're one of the best. Walking away from your job doesn't just hurt you—it hurts the patients who still need you."

Jonathan looked down at his hands again. They felt heavier than they ever had before. "I can't hold a scalpel again knowing what I've done."

The break room faded.

Darkness swallowed the walls, pressing in on him. The hum of the hospital dulled into silence.

And then—light. A single, focused beam illuminated him like a lone figure on a stage.

Except he wasn't alone.

Another Jonathan stepped forward from the shadows. His posture was rigid, his expression hard, and his eyes penetrating.

"You're afraid," the other Jonathan said.

Jonathan barely breathed. "Of course, I am," he replied.

"Fear has no place in the OR."

"That's not true." His voice wavered. Then strengthened. "Fear is what makes me cautious. Fear makes me think before I cut."

"Fear makes you hesitate," the other Jonathan shot back. "It makes you weak."

"No." Jonathan lifted his chin. "It makes me human."

Silence stretched between them, thick and charged.

Jonathan’s gaze didn’t waver. “But without you, I would never make the first cut. I would never take the risk.”

The other Jonathan studied him for a long moment. Then he nodded. “And without you, I wouldn’t know when to stop.”

The space between them shrank.

“We need each other,” Jonathan murmured. “The surgeon who hesitates and the one who charges ahead" The one who fears and the one who acts with conviction.”

There was a whisper of movement, the shifting of shadows.

“We were never meant to be apart,” the other Jonathan said softly.

They stepped toward each other, the gap between them dissolving, until there was no space left at all.

The darkness shattered.

The hospital hum returned. The beeping of monitors resumed. The sound of distant voices filled the air. The break room came back into focus, and Jonathan regained his senses, the weight of the moment settling over him.

Pierce was still watching him, wary. "You okay?"

Jonathan flexed his fingers, feeling the weight of his hands.

They trembled. Then steadied.

"I don't know," he admitted. Then he took a deep breath, and his chest felt lighter. "But I will be."

Pierce didn't reply, just glanced at him sideways.

Jonathan straightened his shoulders. "Tell the chief I'm scrubbing in."

Pierce's lips quirked into the smallest hint of a smile. "Damn right, you are."

Jonathan nodded once, then pushed open the break room door. The fluorescent light of the hallway bathed him in something new.

Not just weight. Not just fear.

Conviction.

And for the first time since the surgery, he knew—his hands were still his own.

They were ready.

And steady.

6. The Sound of Broken Glass

Two doctors discuss the qualities of an exceptional leader.

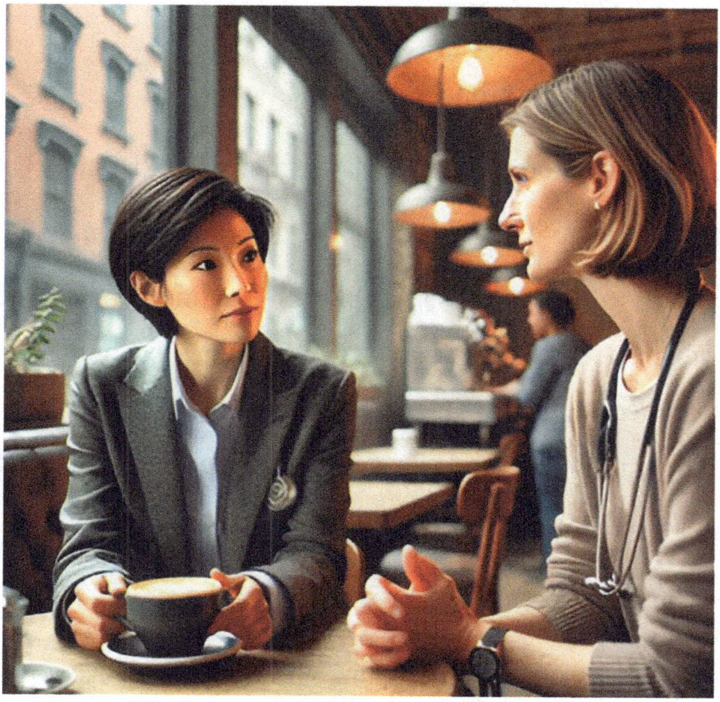

The café was quiet, the warm hum of conversation blending with the hiss of the espresso machine. Dr. Elaine Cheung stirred her tea absently, eyes fixed on the swirling liquid. Across from her, Dr. Mara Westover took a sip of her coffee and stared back.

"You're doing it again."

Elaine glanced up. “Doing what?”

“That thing where you stare into your cup of coffee like it holds the answer to life’s biggest questions.”

Elaine paused as she set down her spoon. “I applied for the CEO position.”

Mara grinned. “About damn time.”

“Don’t get too excited,” Elaine muttered. “I doubt I’ll even get a second look.”

Mara rolled her eyes. “Oh, for—Elaine, you’re the smartest person I know" You practically built that practice. Half the infrastructure changes? Your ideas. The improved workflow? Your implementation. And let’s not forget—”

“I’m a radiologist.”

Mara leaned back, folding her arms. “Ah, here we go.”

Elaine sighed. “Be honest. When you think of a CEO, do you think of someone who spends their day in a dark room, staring at images?”

“I think of someone who solves problems, makes critical decisions, and understands the bigger picture.”

Elaine snorted. “Nice pun.”

“Unintentional,” Mara smirked. “But accurate.”

“You know what I mean,” Elaine said. “CEOs are charismatic, decisive, and out in the trenches. People look up to them. They don’t…analyze shadows on a screen.”

“Right, because catching a pancreatic tumor a year before symptoms develop isn’t dynamic at all.”

Elaine didn’t answer. Instead, she glanced out the window, watching the slow stream of pedestrians moving past. “It’s not just that,” she said after a moment. “You know what they’re thinking. She’s a woman. She’s Asian. She’s a radiologist. For Pete’s sake, Mara, I’m just a doctor. They probably want a Harvard MBA. Better yet, a doctor with a Harvard MBA.”

Mara scoffed. “Oh, please. Half those Harvard MBAs wouldn’t know the first thing about patient care. You know what they know? Spreadsheets and ‘value propositions.’”

Elaine giggled. “And networking. Don’t forget networking.”

Mara grinned. “Right. Because knowing which donor to schmooze is apparently more important than knowing how a health system actually runs.” She bent forward. “You’ve spent twenty years in the trenches. You know the medicine. You know the people. You know what works and what doesn’t. You think a business degree from Harvard is a substitute for that?”

Elaine shook her head. “No.”

Mara nodded. “Then stop acting like you’re applying for a job you don’t deserve. Those MBAs? They should be intimidated by you.”

Elaine let that sit for a moment.

Mara tilted her head. “Unless, of course, you want some guy in a $2,000 suit who’s never touched a stethoscope making decisions about your hospital.”

Elaine smirked. “God, no.”

“Then you know what to do.”

Mara raised her voice. “You know you’re the most competent person for the job.”

"Maybe. But leadership isn't just about competence. It's about…perception. About presence. And I don't know if I have that."

"Do you really believe that?"

Elaine hesitated. "I don't know."

Mara shook her head. "Elaine, leadership isn't about shouting the loudest in a boardroom. It's not about chest-thumping. It's about seeing patterns before anyone else does. It's about knowing when to act and when to wait. It's about making the call that no one else wants to make. It's about noticing trends and patterns.

Elaine let out a small breath. "That's what I do every day."

"Exactly. You think you're not a leader because you don't fit some outdated mold? Elaine, those guys in the running—most of them got here by playing politics. But you? You led by example. You made the tough calls without a fancy title. You are a leader."

Elaine leaned back in her chair, fingers wrapped around the warmth of her cup. "Maybe I just don't feel… whole enough for the job. Like I'm missing something."

"You're looking at the situation all wrong," Mara said. "Leadership isn't about being whole. It's about balancing strength and vulnerability. Your hesitation? It's not weakness; it's awareness. And that's what makes you better than the rest."

Elaine met her gaze, something shifting in her expression. "You really think I have a shot?"

"I think they'd be fools not to pick you."

Elaine smirked. "Well, fools do love their glass ceilings."

Mara raised her cup in a toast. "Then it's time to crack the glass."

Elaine clinked her cup against Mara's, the quiet chime of ceramic punctuating the moment. Outside, the city hummed with possibility.

7. Commander-in-Chief

A psychiatrist attempts to change the mindset of a disruptive physician.

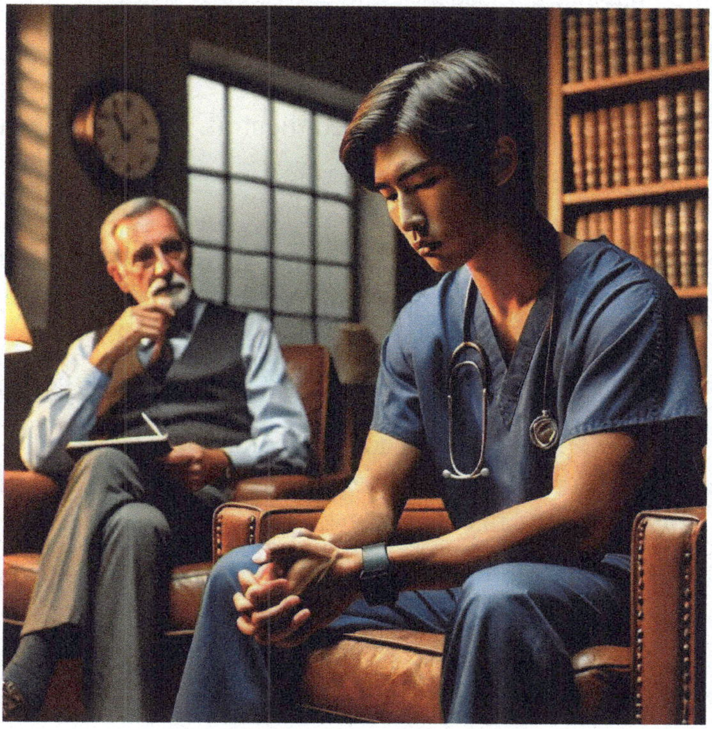

Dr. Eric Sato sat in the leather chair, hands folded, his jaw tight. The psychiatrist's office was dimly lit, the bookshelves lined with dense medical and psychology texts. A clock on the wall ticked steadily, filling the silence between them.

Dr. Bruce Felder, the psychiatrist, sat across from him, legs crossed, a yellow legal pad resting on his knee. He had said nothing for a full minute, simply observing.

Eric exhaled slowly. “So, how does this work? You tell me I have anger issues. I nod and say I’ll work on it, and we all go home happy?”

Felder’s expression remained neutral. “Why do you think you’re here?”

Eric grunted. “Because my department chair has thin skin.”

Felder raised an eyebrow. “And the nursing staff? The residents? The faculty who filed complaints?”

Eric shifted in his seat, his fingers tapping against his knee. “They don’t like my style. I push people to be better—to move faster—and to do their damn jobs. Since when is that a crime?”

Felder jotted something down. “You’re a trauma surgeon.”

Eric nodded. “That’s right.”

“High stakes. Split-second decisions. Life and death, every day.”

Eric's slight frame heaved forward. "Exactly. You hesitate in my OR; people die. You're soft; people die. That's why I push. If that makes me 'disruptive,' then fine."

Felder tapped his pen against his pad. "And you think the best way to ensure success is through…force?"

Eric narrowed his eyes. "Not force. Command. I know what needs to happen. I know what works. And I won't apologize for being direct."

Felder let the silence stretch again. Eric had learned in medical school that silence was a technique, a way to get patients to fill the void. He hated being on this side of it.

Finally, Felder spoke. "Who taught you that being in command is about dominance?"

Eric blinked. "What?"

"You're smart, Dr. Sato. You made it through med school, residency, and fellowship. Somewhere along the way, you decided the only way to command was to be…" Felder gestured vaguely, "this."

Eric's fingers curled into fists. "You don't get it. I have to be like this."

"Why?"

"Because no one listens otherwise! Because if you're weak, they walk all over you. If you hesitate, if you doubt—" He stopped, exhaling deeply.

Felder stared at him. "What happens if you doubt?"

Eric's voice dropped. "You fail."

"And?"

Eric's throat tightened. "People die."

Felder nodded, as if he had expected this answer. "And if you show compassion?"

Eric hesitated.

Felder pushed on. "If you admit uncertainty? If you guide instead of command? If you trust instead of control?"

"Then I become one of those weak, indecisive doctors who never take charge. The ones who overthink, who let patients crash while they debate differentials. Or the ones who pursue medicine from a distance—like you."

Ah! There it was. The type of insult Felder had been trained for. One that has its roots in countertransference.

But Felder knew better than to defend himself. He remained silent, composed. Then, in a calm voice, he asked, "And what if you're wrong—about me—and yourself?"

Eric made a fist again. "I'm not," he said, pounding the arm of his chair.

"You are." Felder retorted, this time raising his voice.

Eric's head snapped up.

Felder's voice remained loud but steady. "Because being in command isn't about being the brassiest, the strongest, or the fastest. It's about balance. Control. But not the kind you think."

Eric swallowed hard.

Felder continued. "You believe strength comes from shutting out doubt. From silencing any part of yourself that hesitates or questions. But you forget—those instincts are also what make you good at what you do. What makes you human?"

Eric looked away.

Felder softened his tone. "You're not just a blade, Dr. Sato. You're also the hand that holds it."

Something inside Eric twisted.

Felder watched him carefully. “There’s a part of you that knows when to push. But there’s also a part that knows when to pull back. You’ve buried that part. You think it’s weakness.”

Eric gulped.

Felder tilted his head. “But what if it isn’t?”

Eric’s mood changed. He became pensive.

For years, he had convinced himself that hesitation, kindness, and patience were just different words for failure. That surgeons had to be cold, unshakable, immune to fear. But now—

What if he had been wrong?

Felder let the silence sway over them, then said quietly, “You’re here because people respect your skill, but they fear you. You can be the surgeon they need and the commander they follow.”

Eric finally met his gaze. “And if I can’t?”

Felder leaned back, his expression unreadable. “Then you’re just a man wielding a knife.”

The words hit deeper than Eric expected. He wasn't a wild man, he thought— not some violent, stark-raving lunatic. But that's just how Felder painted him to be.

A long moment passed. Then, slowly, he looked down at his hands.

They were steady. Strong. Capable.

For the first time, he felt something else.

Responsibility.

Control.

Balance.

Finally, he looked back up. "So, how do I fix this?"

Felder smiled slightly. "You don't fix it. You integrate it."

He explained, "The strength of your command may lie in your darker, disruptive side. In that sense, you're no different than anyone else. We all have our darker side. We need it! It's half of what we are. Call it hostility, lust, violence, or whatever—but it's your positive side, your compassion, love, and tenderness, which you repress, that controls your darker side and makes you a doctor—a teacher and a healer."

Eric nodded.

For the first time in a long time, he didn't feel like a blade. He realized that being a great surgeon is not just about being sharp—it's about knowing when to wield that sharpness and when to step back, knowing when to act, when to push forward, and when to hold back.

Now, Eric felt like the one who knew when to use the scalpel and how to integrate his two halves: the aggressive, commanding surgeon and the reflective, conscientious healer.

It's not just about cutting, he thought as he left Felder's office—it's about understanding when intervention is necessary and when restraint is just as important.

8. Checkmate

A doctor discusses a medical breakthrough, but it means nothing if patients can't afford it.

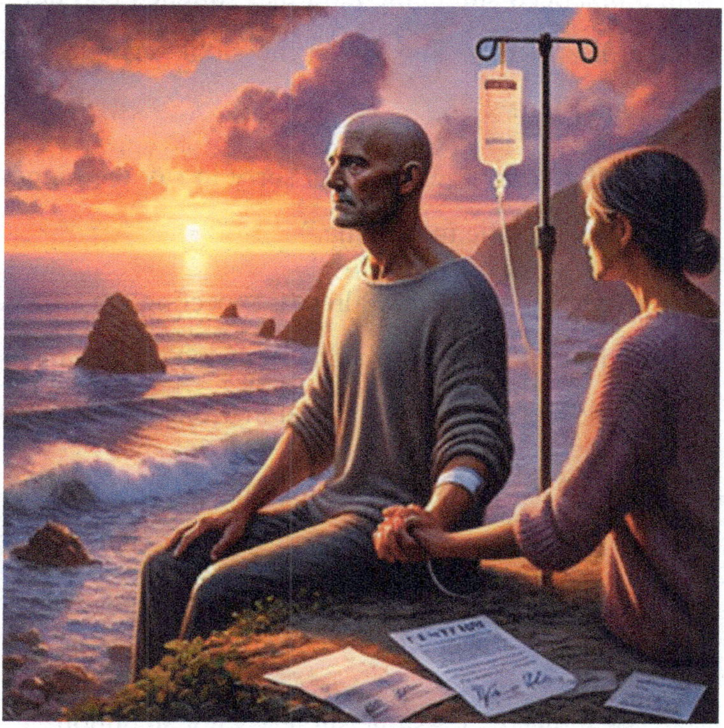

The scent of saltwater clung to Mark Peterson's skin as he stepped into the office. It was an unusually warm afternoon for February on the West Coast, but the chill inside Dr. Leina'ala Keawe's dermatology clinic felt like a different climate altogether. His wife, Emily, sat beside him, her fingers laced tightly through his. The paper crinkled beneath him as he shifted on the exam table. He had always hated the way those disposable sheets made patients feel temporary.

Dr. Keawe, her dark hair glistening with silver, entered with a practiced smile, the kind that softened bad news but never erased it. She sat on the stool, scanning his electronic chart.

“Mark,” she began gently. “I’m sorry to say the biopsy confirms metastatic melanoma.”

Emily let out a sob. Mark, already expecting the words, appeared emotionless. He had spent too many nights with WebMD, tracing the dark trail from a suspicious mole to the unthinkable.

Dr. Keawe steered the stool forward. “I want you to know this: it is not a death sentence. It's not as dire as before.”

Mark swallowed. “I assume surgery’s not an option?”

She shook her head. “It spread. But we have something we didn’t have when I was in training. Something that’s changing everything.”

She stood, pulling a laminated chart from her bookshelf, laying it on the counter. Nivolumab. Ipilimumab. PD-1 inhibitors. CTLA-4 blockade. The words blurred as she spoke.

"Your immune system," she explained, "has brakes—checkpoints—that keep it from attacking your body. But cancer exploits these brakes, making your T-cells—your attack cells—ignore it." She tapped the chart. "These drugs release those brakes. They tell your immune system to see the cancer and fight."

Mark exhaled. "And it works?"

Dr. Keawe nodded. "Ten years ago, a study called CheckMate 067 started tracking patients like you. The ones who got both nivolumab and ipilimumab had a median survival of over six years. Some are still alive today."

Mark felt Emily squeeze his hand. Six years. That was something. That was more sunsets over the Pacific, more birthdays, and more hikes with his son, Daniel. More life.

Then the other shoe dropped.

"How much?" Mark asked.

Dr. Keawe hesitated. "It's expensive."

"How expensive?"

She sighed. "The first year alone—around three hundred thousand."

Emily gasped. Mark let out a dry laugh.

"Checkmate," he muttered.

Dr. Keawe tilted her head.

He gestured vaguely toward the chart. "The trial. CheckMate 067. Funny name, isn't it? A breakthrough treatment, a lifeline—and yet, for most people, it's still a losing game."

Dr. Keawe's voice softened. "I won't pretend this is fair. It isn't. But there are grants, clinical trials—"

Mark shook his head. "I don't have time to play the lottery with trials. We'll find a way."

Emily turned to him, eyes brimming. "Mark, we can't—"

"We'll refinance," he said firmly. "It's just money."

Emily pressed her lips together but said nothing.

Dr. Keawe watched them, sadness in her gaze. "I've seen patients do this," she admitted. "Mortgage their future for a shot at having one."

Mark smiled grimly. “Lucky I have a house.” He ran a hand over his face. “What happens to the ones who don’t?”

* * *

The infusions started the following month. Mark sat for hours in a recliner at the cancer center, watching the IV drip its chemical soldiers into his bloodstream. The side effects came fast—fatigue, nausea, a rash that spread over his arms. His immune system was waking up, and it was angry.

At sunset, he and Emily would walk to the cliffs near their home, watching the sky turn molten over the Pacific. Every evening, he told himself, One more.

Three months in, his first scan showed the tumors shrinking.

Six months in, he had a new, positive obsession with his health.

The waiting room was filled with people just like him—fighters, survivors, but not all of them had the means. He met a man who had been denied coverage. A woman who had to crowdfund her treatment.

And Mark—who had considered himself lucky—felt something shift inside him.

* * *

It started with a letter.

Then another.

Then a petition.

Soon, Mark was standing in the office of his congressman, telling his story. Telling their stories. "These drugs exist," he said, voice steady. "But what good is a miracle if only a few can afford it?"

The movement grew. News outlets picked it up. Policy discussions began.

Mark kept fighting.

And every evening, as the sun melted into the horizon, he held Emily's hand and whispered to himself:

One more.

And then another.

And another.

9. Medicine's Internecine War

"A house divided against itself cannot stand." — Abraham Lincoln

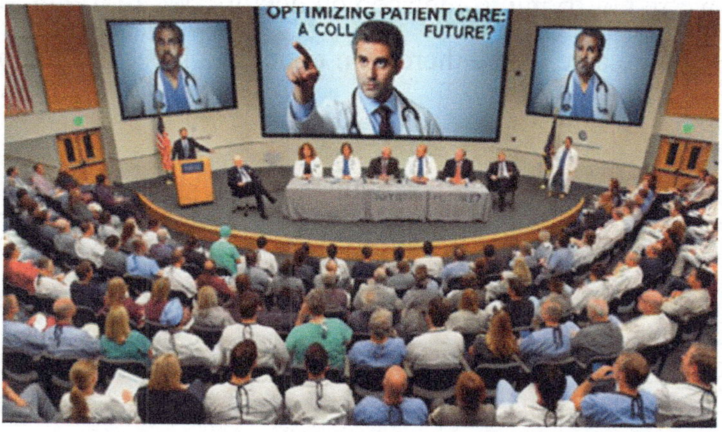

The auditorium buzzed with restless energy at the quarterly all-staff meeting at Oakridge Medical Center. Physicians, NPs, PAs, CRNAs, pharmacists, and hospital administrators were present—some with arms crossed, others tapping pens against notepads. A PowerPoint slide behind the podium read:

"Optimizing Patient Care: A Collaborative Future?"

No one had any illusions—this was about to turn into a turf war.

Dr. Alan Bishop, a grizzled internal medicine physician with three decades under his belt, leaned back in his chair. “Let’s go at it,” he muttered.

Jane Nguyen, a seasoned NP, began. “Respectfully, we’re not trying to replace you doctors. We’re trying to provide care where there aren’t enough physicians to do it.”

Dr. Robert Cahill, a hospitalist, gave a short laugh, his voice edged with irritation. “That’s the line we keep hearing, Jane. But let’s talk numbers. APPs claim they’re filling physician shortages, but workforce data shows something different. Many aren’t setting up shop in rural areas at all—they're in cities, competing with us for the same insured patients.”

A murmur spread through the room.

Dr. Deepa Patel, a primary care physician, nodded. “And when hospitals push to expand NP and PA privileges, it’s not out of some noble mission to serve the underserved—it’s because APPs are cheaper hires. Let’s be honest: this is about economics, not access.”

Jane felt a lump in her throat. “It’s not that simple. Not all of us want to work in rural areas. Frankly, some of your colleagues also refuse to practice there. Should we just let patients suffer?"

"Of course not," Cahill shot back. "But you can't claim you're fixing a shortage when you're flooding metro areas. And let's be clear: the solution isn't substituting four years of medical school, three to seven years of residency, a fellowship, and board exams with a two-year master's degree and online clinical hours."

A few gasps were heard. Someone muttered, "Oh, boy."

Dr. Thomas Greer, an orthopedic surgeon, became emotional. "If we're going to talk about encroachment, let's talk about it across the board. Podiatrists are pushing for surgical privileges to operate on ankles. If that happens, what's stopping optometrists from performing eye surgery? Or chiropractors from managing back fractures?"

Dr. Norma Chang, a podiatrist, stiffened. "Are you suggesting podiatrists aren't qualified to handle foot and ankle issues? We train for this, Dr. Greer. More than you give us credit for."

Greer smirked. "Surgical residency matters. Cadaver labs matter. You can't compare a three-year podiatric program to an orthopedic surgical residency. And yet, hospital administrators keep trying to blur those lines."

The room whirred with tension.

Lisa Warren, a CRNA, came forward. "With all due respect, this kind of infighting is exactly why hospitals, insurers, and corporate medicine take advantage of us. We should be fighting the real problem—the middlemen in suits who dictate reimbursement, limit access to care, and devalue all of us."

A rare silence settled.

Dr. Patel exhaled. "Lisa's right. We're clawing at each other while the real power brokers profit from the chaos."

At the far end of the table, David Langston, the hospital's CFO, cleared his throat and began to speak. "I take issue with that characterization. We're all in this together. We don't set reimbursement rates—insurance companies do. And we certainly don't control physician training pipelines or rural shortages. We have to work with the resources we have. If we only hired physicians, we couldn't stay solvent."

Dr. Cahill turned toward Langston, eyebrows raised. "You couldn't stay solvent? The CEO's salary just hit $5 million last year. How many primary care physicians could you hire with that?"

Langston frowned. "That's a separate issue."

"Is it?" Patel shot back. "Because the number of non-clinical hospital administrators has ballooned over the past decade, while we've seen cuts to staffing, reduced physician salaries, and increased workload. You're running this place like a corporation, not a hospital."

Langston sighed. "Look, hospitals don't make the rules. We have to deal with the realities of Medicare cuts, commercial insurance negotiations, and financial constraints. If we don't use Advanced Practice Providers (APPs), and if we don't make strategic hiring decisions, we will have to close departments and limit patient care."

Cahill snapped, "You mean ration patient care."

Dr. Martin Rowe, the hospital's Chief Medical Officer (CMO), interjected. "Then let's talk real solutions instead of pointing fingers. First, scope of practice needs clearer boundaries — not dictated by lobbying groups, but by training, case volume, and patient outcomes.

Physicians should lead care teams. APPs should complement, not substitute."

Greer glanced at Chang. "And surgical privileges should be based on residency training and case complexity—not just how many procedures a lobbying board says someone should do."

Chang gave a slow nod. "If that's applied across all disciplines, I'd accept that."

Patel raised a hand. "And we need physician-led policy reform. Every time hospitals cut MDs and DOs in favor of APPs, it's because insurers and hospital boards see clinicians as a 'cost center.' We should be driving policy—not corporate executives who've never seen a patient."

Langston shook his head. "That's easier said than done. You're talking about upending the entire financial model of modern healthcare."

Rowe's lips curled into a wry smile. "No, we're talking about returning medical decision-making to those actually practicing medicine."

There was a long pause.

Dr. Cahill smirked. “Well, I’ll be damned. Maybe we don’t need divine intervention after all.”

Langston sat back, silent. He wasn’t going to win this fight.

The meeting adjourned. No one held hands and sang Kumbaya, but at least, for once, they weren’t about to throw daggers at one another. Instead, they had finally found their common enemy.

10. A Matter of Instinct

Ignoring a doctor's judgment and blindly adhering to a protocol leads to a tragedy.

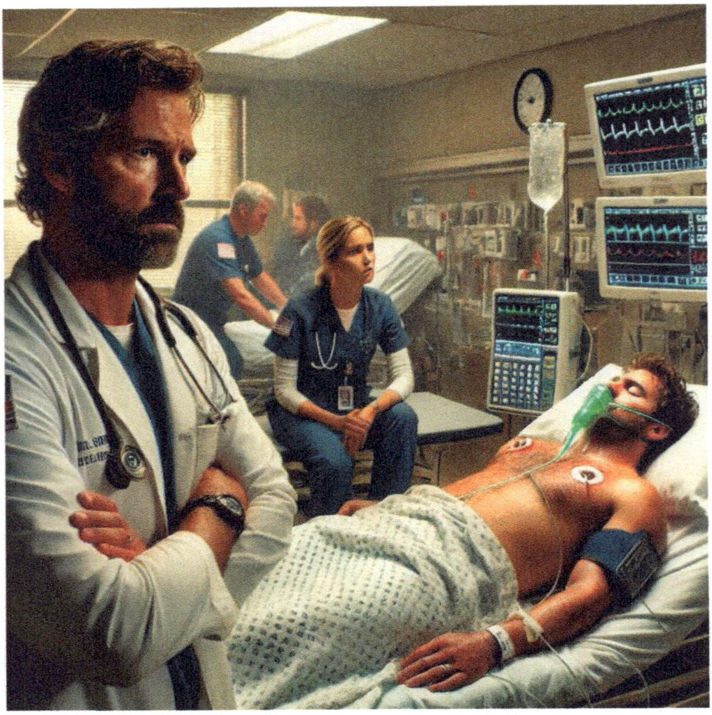

"ETA ten minutes. The patient is a male in his early forties. Severe anaphylaxis. CPR in progress," the radio crackled.

Dr. Ben Whitaker wiped his forehead and braced himself. The air in the tiny five-bed ER of Garson County General had a whiff of alcohol wipes and sterile gauze. This was his weekend alone, covering everything from heart attacks to calf-roping injuries.

“Damn,” murmured Ellie, the night nurse. “We’re flying blind without an allergist around.”

“We’re flying, period,” Ben muttered.

When the paramedics burst through the double doors, the patient’s face was grotesquely swollen, his skin the color of bruised peaches. The rhythm strip on the monitor showed a pulseless electrical activity—PEA arrest.

“Name’s Christopher Langley,” one of the paramedics said between breaths. “Severe reaction, unknown allergen. Epi on arrival, no response. Twenty minutes down. We’ve been bagging him.”

Ben examined him quickly. The distorted airway was beyond recognition. Not just swollen—wooden. A classic case of what textbooks warned against: the kind of airway no tube could navigate.

“Ellie, one milligram of epinephrine IV push,” Ben ordered, knowing it was a long shot. He pressed two fingers to the patient’s neck. Nothing.

“You’re thinking cricothyrotomy?” Ellie asked.

“Has to be,” Ben said. “Scalpel, bougie, and a 6.0 ET tube.”

A nurse handed him the scalpel. The room became eerily quiet. Ben made a single incision at the cricothyroid membrane, sliding the tube in with precision. He felt the telltale sign of entry, then the rush of air.

“Bag him.”

Ellie squeezed the Ambu bag, and the O_2 sats crawled up. A heartbeat flickered on the monitor.

“He's back,” Ellie whispered.

Ben nodded, but something felt wrong. Christopher’s pulse was there, but weak. His blood pressure wobbled at 68/40. The usual protocol called for more fluids and more pressors. But Ben hesitated.

Something about this was...different. The standard treatment wasn’t working. His gut, that instinct honed by years of watching patients teeter on the brink, told him that pushing too hard with fluids could drown his fragile circulation.

He pivoted. “Lower the IV fluids. Keep the epi drip running, but at a slower rate.”

A beat. Then two. The numbers stabilized. Not perfect, but holding.

Ellie exhaled. "Whew, you did it."

"We did it," Ben corrected.

The whine of rotor blades signaled the arrival of the medi-vac team. Two flight medics strode in, all crisp uniforms and clipped efficiency.

"What've we got?" the taller one asked.

Ben met his eyes. "Critical anaphylaxis, but listen to me carefully—his vascular tone is fragile. Too much fluid or an aggressive pressor push will collapse him."

The medics nodded, the kind of nod people give when they've already made up their minds.

Ben's stomach twisted. He grabbed the lead medic's arm. "I mean it. Do not overload him. Keep him exactly where he is."

Another nod. Another lie.

They wheeled Christopher out.

* * *

Ben called the university hospital the next morning.

"He didn't make it," the ICU attending said flatly. "Crashed in flight. Hypotension, cardiac arrest. They couldn't get him back."

Ben closed his eyes. "What did they do?"

"They gave him two liters of fluids and doubled his epi drip en route."

A hollow silence stretched between them.

Ben hung up.

Ellie found him an hour later, staring at the ER doors. "You're not okay."

He shook his head, voice brittle. "I knew it. I told them. And they killed him anyway."

She didn't try to offer comfort. There wasn't any.

Later that day, Ben called the medivac team. When the lead medic answered, he didn't bother with pleasantries.

"I told you exactly what to do."

There was a long pause in the conversation. Then, a defensive voice said, "We followed standard protocol."

Ben's voice turned to steel. "Your protocol killed him."

Silence.

Then, the weak excuse: "We had to make a judgment call."

Ben's fingers tightened around the phone. "No. You didn't. I made the call. You ignored it."

The silence stretched.

Then, the medic said, "Look, Doc, these things happen—"

Ben hung up.

He sat for a long time, staring at nothing.

Then he stood, turned, and went back to work.

11. The Detective

A doctor follows the clues and asks the right questions to prevent the trail from growing cold.

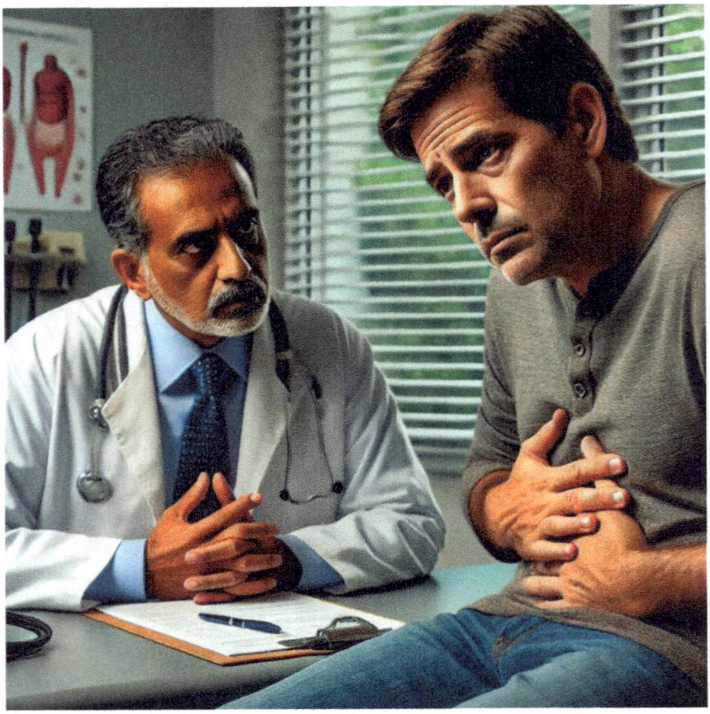

Dr. Rajan Varma had a reputation in the community for being a kind and compassionate gastroenterologist, never in a rush, and certainly never prone to turning away difficult cases. His fingers interlaced as he questioned the man across from him. Forty-two years old, average overweight, eyes rimmed with exhaustion.

The chart labeled him simply as John Matthews, Chronic Abdominal Pain—Unresolved.

Dr. Varma had read between the lines. The multiple referrals. The unhelpful tests. The unspoken frustration persists.

"Doctor, I just need the issue fixed," John groaned. "My stomach's a wreck. Feels like knives twisting. And no one can figure out why."

"I read your history." Dr. Varma said, elbows resting on his desk. "You've seen your primary care doctor, a cardiologist, and even a surgeon, correct?"

"Yeah. My PCP thought it might be my gallbladder or heart-related—something he called "atypical cardiac pain." They ran tests—EKG, stress test, even a CT scan of my abdomen. Everything's fine, they said.".

Dr. Varma tapped his pen. "Tell me about your job."

"Software engineer."

"Hours?"

"Fifty, sometimes sixty a week. But this isn't stress, Doc. It's physical."

"Where are you from originally?"

John squinted. "Grew up in Iowa."

Dr. Varma smiled. "What did you eat growing up? Home-cooked or processed?"

John shrugged. "Mom cooked. Basic midwest fare—meatloaf, mashed potatoes, pork chops."

"And now?"

"Mostly takeout. I don't have much time to cook.

Dr. Varma's fingers drummed the desk. Something nagged at him. He had seen this pattern before, back in his home country, when a woman had suffered for months with vague stomach pains before someone figured it out.

He took a different approach. "Ever travel outside the U.S.?"

John blinked. "Uh… yeah, three months ago. Work sent me to Vietnam."

Dr. Varma's eyes sharpened. "You had a trip abroad, and a month later, you developed pain?"

"Well, yeah, but the symptoms started slow."

Dr. Varma straightened. "John, has anyone checked you for strongyloidiasis?"

John's face twisted in confusion. "Strongylo—what?"

"A parasitic infection. A parasitic infection can remain undetected for years. Many doctors don't test for it because it's rare here. But in Southeast Asia and some other parts of the world, it's not. Some cases present exactly like yours—chronic abdominal pain with no clear cause."

John sat up. "Are you serious? You think I have a parasite?"

"I think it's possible. And if it is, a simple medication could solve a mystery that's plagued you for months."

John hesitated, then grinned wryly. "So, what—you're like a medical Sherlock Holmes?"

Dr. Varma chuckled. "More like a detective who listens. The clues were always there."

Two weeks later, John returned, shaking his head in disbelief.

"You were right," he said. "The test came back positive. One dose of ivermectin, and I feel like a new man."

Dr. Varma smiled. He had spent years adapting to American medicine—learning its strengths and its blind spots. Some things, though, were universal.

A good doctor always follows the trail.

12. A Shot for Everything

A doctor's quick fix doesn't necessarily provide long-term solutions.

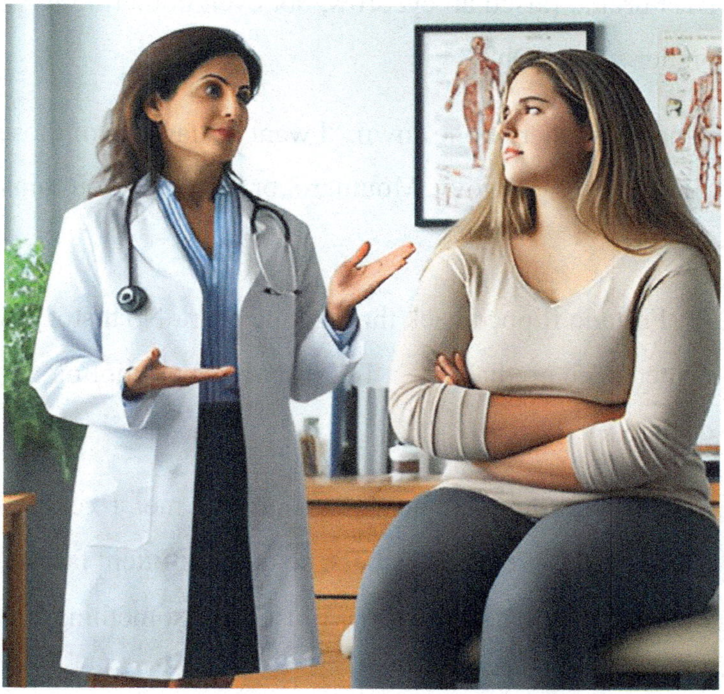

Dr. Ana Furtado sighed as she skimmed the patient chart before stepping into the exam room. Amanda Tate, 42 years old. BMI: 38. Complaint: "Request for weight loss medication."

She knew the conversation before it even started.

Inside, Amanda was perched on the edge of the exam table, scrolling on her phone. She looked up and smiled. "Hey, Doc. I know why I'm here, and I promise I won't take up much of your time."

Dr. Furtado raised an eyebrow, not even bothering to sit on her stool. "Oh?"

Amanda set her phone down. "I want to start one of those GLP-1 shots. Wegovy, Mounjaro, or whatever you think is best."

Dr. Furtado flipped back through the chart. No history of diabetes, no prediabetes. "Tell me what's prompting this decision."

Amanda gestured at herself. "Look at me. I've tried everything—Weight Watchers, keto, intermittent fasting. I lose; I gain. I'm tired, Doc. I just want something that works."

Dr. Furtado stepped forward. "Let's talk about your daily routine. Walk me through a typical day—meals, movement, sleep."

Amanda groaned. "Ugh. Do we have to? I work full-time, I have two kids, and my husband's schedule is insane. I eat when I can. Most days, it's takeout or something quick. I'm not gonna pretend I have time for home-cooked meals."

Dr. Furtado nodded. "Exercise?"

Amanda waved a dismissive hand. "I mean, I run around all day. That counts, right?"

Dr. Furtado paused, choosing her words carefully. "Amanda, these medications work best with lifestyle changes. They're not a magic bullet."

Amanda frowned. "But I've heard people lose fifty, sixty pounds on them."

"They can help, but they don't replace movement, nutrition, or sleep. And they have side effects—nausea, vomiting, and muscle loss if you're not eating enough protein."

Amanda crossed her arms. "But it's FDA-approved. Insurance should cover it. What's the big deal?"

Dr. Furtado hesitated. She could hear the frustration beneath Amanda's words.

"The big deal," she said gently, "is that we're treating obesity like an infection, something to be 'fixed' with a prescription. But weight isn't just biology. It's about stress, access to healthy food, time, movement, and sleep—all the things our medical system doesn't fix."

Amanda was annoyed. "So, what, I'm supposed to just eat salad and jog every day?"

Dr. Furtado shook her head. "I'm saying we shouldn't pretend weight is just a medication problem. If we don't address the real issues—stress, food access, sleep—you'll regain the weight when you stop the medication. That's what happens to most people. I want you to succeed long-term."

Amanda was silent.

Finally, she muttered, "So you won't prescribe it?"

Dr. Furtado leaned back. "Let's work on small, realistic changes first. If we make progress and you still want the medication in a few months, we can reconsider. But I won't just hand you a prescription and pretend that's the solution."

Amanda stared at the floor. "I just… I don't want to be stuck like this forever."

Dr. Furtado softened. "I know. And I want to help. But not with false promises. Let's really get you healthy."

Amanda sighed. "Fine. What's first?"

Dr. Furtado smiled. Step one: breaking the cycle of quick fixes.

13. The Third Hand

A doctor is guided by unseen forces, revealing the mystery of healing.

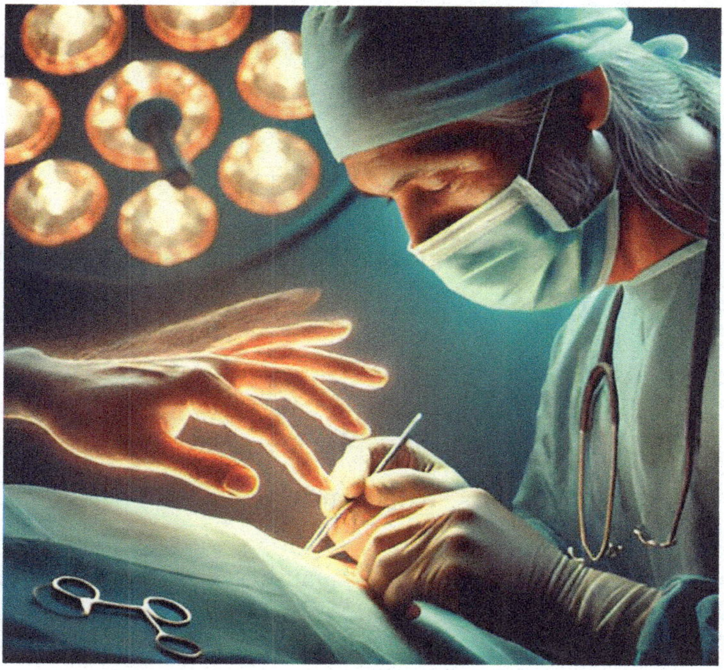

"Dr. Kanoa, are you ready?"

Dr. Micah Kanoa exhaled slowly, rolling his shoulders back as he stepped into the pre-op area. The anxious energy was palpable. He had performed hundreds of surgeries—too many to count—but tonight felt different. Heavy.

On the gurney before him lay Mr. Woodward, a retired schoolteacher in his late sixties. The nurses had finished prepping him, his frail body engulfed in crisp white sheets. His wife, Celia, stood by his side, holding his hand, whispering words too soft for anyone else to hear.

Dr. Kanoa cleared his throat. “Mr. Woodward, we’re going to take good care of you.”

Woodward nodded weakly. “I trust you, Doc.”

Celia’s eyes, deep pools of both faith and fear, met Micah’s. “Doctor… I just want you to know we've been praying. For you, too.”

Micah offered a tight smile. He had heard this before. “I appreciate that, Mrs. Woodward.”

She squeezed her husband’s hand one last time before stepping back. The OR doors swung open, swallowing them into the sterile world beyond.

* * *

Inside the operating room, the tension was thick. An abdominal aneurysm. A silent killer. If it ruptured on the table, they’d lose him in minutes.

Dr. Kanoa scrubbed in, methodically working through the routine. Control the artery. Replace the damaged vessel. No room for error.

The problem was, aneurysms had a mind of their own. The pre-op scans were clear—Woodward's had expanded, dangerously thin, a fragile balloon ready to burst. Micah had mapped out the approach, but he also knew surgery wasn't always as simple as a plan on paper.

As the anesthesiologist gave the go-ahead, the room quieted.

Micah made the first incision.

Then it happened.

The aneurysm ruptured instantly, before he could clamp it.

Blood surged, red and unrelenting.

The beeping of the monitors accelerated.

"Suction!" he barked. "Clamp now!"

The scrub nurse handed him the instrument, but his hands weren't steady. He was losing ground.

Not yet. I need time.

For the first time in years, doubt crept in.

He wasn't fast enough. He wasn't good enough. Maybe he never had been.

And then—

A presence.

A shift in the air, like the tide pulling back before a great wave could crash.

Warmth. A certainty not his own.

A still, quiet voice in his mind:

"You are not alone."

His hands steadied. His breath slowed.

He moved with precision—not just skill, but something greater.

In that moment, it wasn't just him holding the clamp, suturing the vessel, restoring the flow. There was a third hand guiding his own.

The bleeding stopped.

The room exhaled.

"He's stabilizing," the anesthesiologist shouts with glee.

Micah stepped back in amazement. The rupture had been catastrophic. The survival odds? Slim. And yet, Mr. Woodward was still here.

* * *

Hours had gone by while Celia sat anxiously in the waiting room.

Dr. Kanoa approached, still wearing his surgical cap. She rose to her feet before he could even speak.

"Mrs. Woodward..." He hesitated. "We lost control for a moment. He shouldn't have made it."

Her eyes welled up. "But he did."

Micah nodded slowly. "He did."

She placed a gentle hand on his arm. "You know why, don't you?"

Micah's throat tightened. He thought back to the presence in the OR, to the moment his fear vanished, to the third hand that had steadied his own.

He had spent his career believing in skill, training, and precision. But maybe...just maybe...that wasn't the whole story.

Celia smiled knowingly. "We prayed for you."

Micah, the man of science, the surgeon with steady hands, the one who always took all the responsibility—

—simply nodded.

And whispered, "I know."

* * *

Later that night, as he stood outside the hospital, absorbing the crisp, cool air in a cloudless night, Micah found himself staring up at the stars. He had been raised on stories of his kūpuna—his ancestors—who believed in unseen forces, in the wisdom of the waves and the whispers of the wind. But having left Oahu many years ago for the mainland, Micah had lost touch with his Hawaiian heritage, a culture where spirituality and reverence for the divine are deeply intertwined with nature and the environment.

His tūtū wahine (grandmother) had once told him, "Ke Akua (The God) does not only guide the fisherman in the ocean. He guides the hands of the healer, too."

He had smiled at the time, dismissing it as the words of an elder who saw the world through the lens of faith. But tonight, under the quiet glow of the stars, he wondered.

Maybe belief wasn't about abandoning science. Maybe it wasn't about choosing between skill and something greater.

Maybe it was about knowing that he was an instrument, not the healer, and there were times when the Almighty did indeed work through doctors.

14. Copy, Paste, Catastrophe

A doctor's lack of critical thinking and real-time reassessment *almost cost a life.*

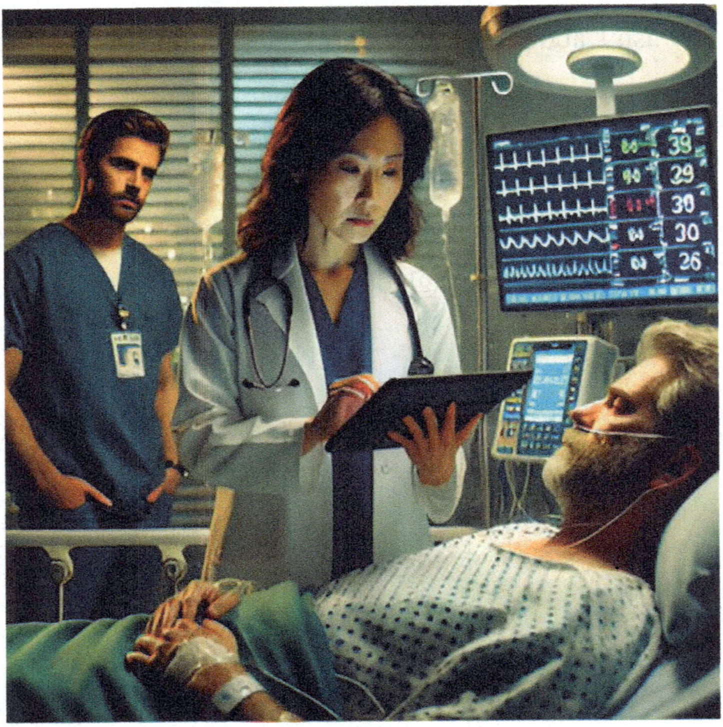

Dr. Xiu Zhang, a hospitalist, strode into the ICU, her coffee untouched and her patience running thin. The rapid response team had been called overnight for a hypotensive crisis—the second one in two days. She had a sinking feeling about what she was about to find.

The patient, Mr. Ray Holloway, lay motionless in his hospital bed, and the monitors were beeping at slow, rhythmic intervals. His BP was barely holding at 92/60. A critical care nurse, Jared, greeted Dr. Zhang at the bedside.

"We almost lost him last night," Jared said, shaking his head. "Again."

Dr. Zhang scanned the electronic chart, her eyes narrowing. "Who was on call?"

"Dr. Lawson, but he followed the plan in the progress note."

She pulled up the latest entry: Day 6—Management of Sepsis.

- Continue IV fluids
- Monitor renal function
- Await nephrology input for worsening creatinine.

Her brow furrowed. The exact same note had appeared for the past five days, word for word.

She clicked on nephrology's consult note. Same thing. Day after day, a copy-pasted assessment:

- “Will reassess in AM.”

Dr. Zhang slammed the tablet onto the counter. “No one changed anything. They just copied and pasted.”

Jared exhaled. “So, what’s the real plan?”

Dr. Zhang threw her arms up. “That’s the problem. There is no plan.”

* * *

An hour later, Dr. Zhang sat across from Dr. Bryan Lawson, a second-year internal medicine resident, grilling him about Mr. Holloway.

“Bryan,” she said slowly, “why did you keep copying the same note for the past five days?”

Dr. Lawson looked flustered. “I— I thought it was just updating the chart. I mean, the attending before I used it, and I figured—”

“You figured the plan was still accurate?”

“Yes. And nephrology followed, so I assumed they’d intervene if needed.”

Dr. Zhang sighed. “You assumed. Bryan, tell me why we kept giving IV fluids.”

"Well, Mr. Holloway was septic, and—"

"He was septic," she corrected. "But the antibiotics worked. He's not hypotensive from infection anymore. He's in fluid overload. That's why we had two rapid responses in 48 hours."

Dr. Lawson's face went pale. "Oh, God."

"Oh, God is right," she snapped. "No one caught it because everyone just copied and pasted the same note. Nephrology didn't change their recommendations, and no one questioned it."

Dr. Lawson's voice was small. "I thought… I thought I was just being efficient."

Dr. Zhang's expression softened. "I know. We all do it. But medicine isn't copy and paste. It's observe, interpret, and act."

Dr. Lawson swallowed. "So, what now?"

Dr. Zhang stood. "Now? We stop fluids, start diuretics, and actually think."

* * *

That evening, Dr. Zhang visited Mr. Holloway's room. He was breathing easier, and the monitors no longer screamed impending doom.

Jared, the nurse, smirked as she checked the vitals. "Amazing what happens when doctors actually change the plan."

Dr. Zhang chuckled. "No more copy, paste, and pray."

Dr. Lawson, standing in the doorway, nodded solemnly. "Lesson learned."

A good doctor doesn't just document the past. A good doctor changes the future.

15. The Anatomy of Doubt

A medical student tries to rid herself of imposter syndrome by listening to her alter ego.

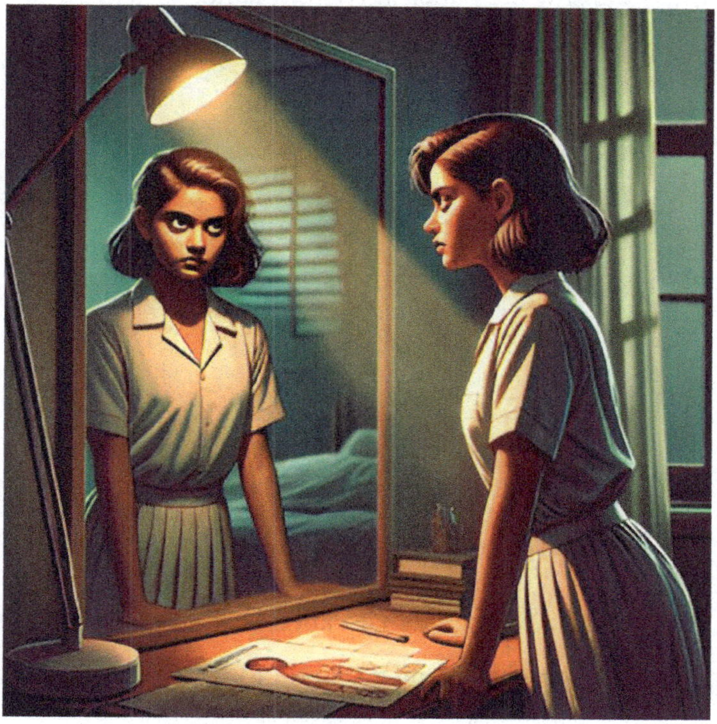

The dorm room was dim, the glow of the desk lamp stretching long shadows across the walls. Nisha sat cross-legged on her bed, her back hunched, fingers gripping the edges of a crumpled anatomy exam. 62%. The number glared up at her, confirming what she had feared all along.

She swallowed hard. "I don't belong here." The words barely made it past her lips.

The door creaked open. Meera walked in, her backpack slung over one shoulder, mid-yawn. She stopped short when she saw the paper in Nisha's hands.

"Oh," she said. "The exam?"

Nisha nodded, silent.

Meera set her bag down, crossing the room. "Well, hey, it's just one test. Anatomy is brutal. Everyone bombs their first—"

"Not everyone."

Meera sighed. "Okay, most people. And even if they didn't, so what?"

"So what?" A bitter laugh escaped Nisha's throat. "I was lucky to even get into med school. I knew I wasn't smart enough, and now I have proof."

Meera sat down next to her. "Nisha…"

"I'm not like you." Nisha shook her head. "You grew up around doctors. You dissected a frog when you were five. I had to Google what the brachial plexus was last week. I don't think like a doctor. I don't have whatever it' is."

Meera leaned back against the headboard, stretching her legs. "You mean imposter syndrome? Because that's what this is."

Nisha looked away. "No, it's not," she murmured. "That would mean I actually deserved to be here. This—this is just realizing the truth."

For a long moment, Meera said nothing. Then she sighed and nudged Nisha's knee with her own. "Look, I could give you the whole pep talk about how you belong here, how you're just as smart as the rest of us, how one test doesn't define you." She shrugged. "And all of that would be true."

Nisha didn't answer.

"But I know you wouldn't believe it," Meera added softly.

Nisha exhaled. "Exactly."

Meera squeezed her shoulder before climbing into bed. "You have to believe it for yourself," she said.

The room fell quiet. Meera's breathing slowed, settling into the steady rhythm of sleep. But Nisha stayed where she was, staring at the test, then setting it aside.

Her gaze drifted to the mirror on the other side of the room. She stood slowly, stepping toward it.

In the dim light, her reflection looked back at her, eyes dark with exhaustion.

“So, this is it?” a voice asked.

Nisha’s breath caught. She looked around, then back at the mirror.

Her reflection smirked. “One bad grade and you quit?”

Nisha blinked. “What—?”

“You know who I am.”

A wave of nausea rolled over her. “Great,” she muttered. “I’ve officially cracked.”

“No,” the reflection said. “You’re just finally listening to yourself. The part of you that doesn’t let fear win.”

“Fear isn’t winning,” Nisha argued. “Reality is.”

The reflection’s head tilted slightly. “Is it?”

Nisha swallowed.

“Because the reality is, you made it into med school. The reality is, you’ve worked just as hard as everyone else here. The reality is, you’re at least their equal.”

"I don't feel like I deserve to be here."

"Feelings aren't facts." The reflection's voice was calm, steady. "If you quit now, you're proving nothing except that you never gave yourself a chance."

Nisha's throat tightened. "But what if I fail again?"

"Then you fail," the reflection said simply. "And you try again. That's the process of becoming a doctor."

Silence stretched between them. Nisha inhaled, long and deep. The reflection gave a small nod, then faded into the glass, leaving only Nisha staring back at herself.

She was alone again. But something felt different.

Her gaze dropped to the exam one last time before she folded it neatly and tucked it away.

The desk lamp clicked off. The room faded to darkness, except for the quiet glow of resolve and the echo of the Dean's words at orientation:

"You all belong here."

16. When Healing Means Comfort and Letting Go

A medical student learns that hospice is not about losing patients—it's about guiding them and their families toward peace.

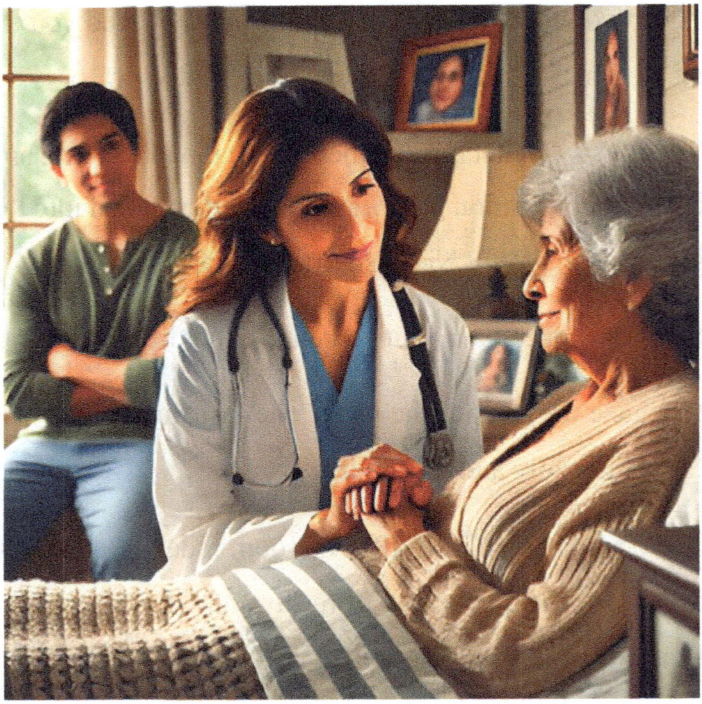

The first thing Luis Domínguez noticed about Dr. Consuelo Martinez was her voice. It wasn't rushed like the surgeons he had shadowed last week. It wasn't tired like the internal medicine residents he had seen drowning in notes. It was steady, almost musical, carrying warmth even when she spoke of difficult things.

They were walking toward the inpatient hospice unit when she asked, "Why hospice?"

Luis hesitated. Why hospice? The truth was, he didn't know. He had rotated through high-energy specialties—emergency medicine, surgery, and critical care. Hospice had felt like a slow lane in comparison. But something about it intrigued him, even if he couldn't explain why.

"I guess… I wanted to experience a slower pace and understand what it means to be a doctor when there's nothing left to fix," he finally said.

Dr. Martinez smiled. "That's a good reason."

***

Their first stop was Mrs. Eliza Contreras, a 79-year-old woman with metastatic ovarian cancer. Her family filled the room—children, grandchildren, even a great-grandchild nestled in a stroller. The air was thick with the smell of vanilla lotion and sadness.

Luis stood by the doorway, watching.

"Eliza, my dear," Dr. Martinez said softly, taking the frail woman's hand. "How are you today?"

Mrs. Contreras blinked, as if waking from a dream. "Tired…but not in pain."

"Good. That means the medication is working."

A son—early 50s, sleeves rolled up—spoke. "Doctor, how much, ugh, longer?"

Dr. Martinez stood firm. Luis felt the weight of the question pressing on the room.

"I think…not much longer," she said gently. "Her breathing is changing. She's comfortable."

The son nodded slowly, his eyes glistening. "We just don't want her to suffer."

"She isn't suffering," Dr. Martinez assured him. "She's still here, still hearing your voices, still feeling your touch."

As they left the room, Luis whispered, "How do you know what to say?"

Dr. Martinez smiled. "I don't always. I just listen."

***

Their next stop was Mr. Gerard Lasky, a 68-year-old stroke patient who had been expected to pass within days. That was two weeks ago.

He lay motionless, eyes open, staring at the ceiling. His wife sat in a chair beside him, wringing her hands, her face drawn with exhaustion.

Dr. Martinez pulled up a chair beside her. "He's holding on."

The woman nodded, eyes filling. "I don't know what to do, Doctor. He was supposed to go peacefully. But now… I sit here every day, waiting."

Dr. Martinez placed a hand on hers. "It's okay to feel that way. You don't have to be ashamed of wanting peace for him."

Mrs. Lasky let out a breath. "I feel like a terrible person for thinking it, but I just want this to be over."

Luis shifted uncomfortably. He had never seen a doctor tell a patient's family that it was okay to want death to come.

Dr. Martinez didn't flinch. "You're not terrible. You're human. And Gerard is leaving on his own time. Not ours."

Mrs. Lasky wiped her tears. "Thank you."

As they stepped out, Luis took a deep breath. "That was…intense."

Dr. Martinez nodded. "Hospice isn't just about the patient, Luis. It's about the people they leave behind."

***

As their day ended, Luis followed Dr. Martinez into her office, still turning everything over in his mind.

"I think I get it now," he admitted.

Dr. Martinez tilted her head. "Get what?"

"Why do you do this work? It's not just about dying. It's about making it okay to die."

She smiled. "Exactly."

Luis hesitated. Because he was bilingual, he had a hunch. "Can I ask…did your parents name you after someone?"

Dr. Martinez laughed. "Not someone. Something. My mother told me that when I was born, she wanted me to bring comfort to others."

Luis understood. He told himself that Consuelo means comfort in Spanish.

"Turns out, she was right," Dr. Martinez remarked.

"I can see that," Luis acknowledged. "Maybe hospice isn't so slow after all."

"The work can be very challenging at times," Dr. Martinez reflected, "but it is also immensely rewarding. Ultimately, what matters most is not the number of patients I lose, but the comfort and care I provide to those nearing the end of their lives. I have come to believe that nothing is more powerful than the love and compassion we can extend to those who are dying. It is a privilege to witness the final moments of a person's life and to assist them in finding peace and dignity as they face death."

Dr. Martinez gathered her things. As she walked down the hall, Luis watched her go. Dr. Consuelo Martinez. The doctor who didn't fight death. The doctor who guided patients—and families—toward it. With comfort.

17. Career Code Blues

Residents resolve not to make medicine more difficult than it already is.

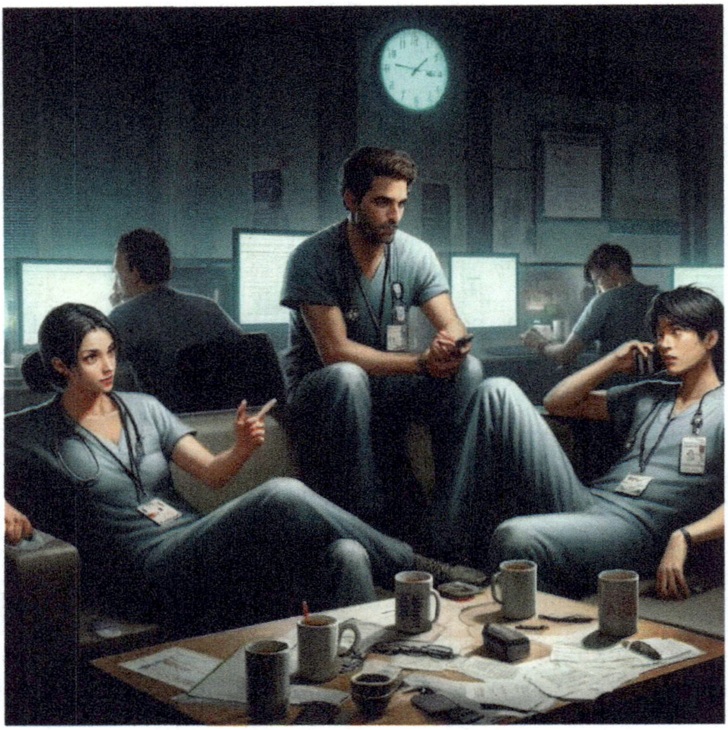

The on-call room smelled like old pizza with a faint hint of lavender from the air freshener someone had opportunistically placed in the corner. Carolyn, Rhett, and Yoichi, three internal medicine residents, sprawled around the room, waiting for their pagers to ruin their peace.

"Okay," Rhett said, stretching his arms behind his head. "Biggest career mistakes doctors make—go."

Carolyn snorted. "Other than picking medicine in the first place?"

Yoichi grinned. "C'mon, let's make it interesting. Not just mistakes, but attendings we've actually heard about screwing up."

Rhett rubbed his hands together. "Oh, I got one. Dr. Potter in Pulmonary."

"You mean the guy who's been at the same hospital for twenty-five years and wonders where his gold watch is?" Carolyn asked.

"That's him," Rhett said. "Apparently, he was offered a leadership role at a big academic center a decade ago but turned it down because, 'This place is family.'"

"Oof," Yoichi cringed.

"Then the hospital merged, admin gutted his department, and suddenly he was just another cog in the machine."

"Or another brick in the wall," Carolyn chimed, in shades of Pink Floyd. "Loyalty's great, but loyalty isn't a retirement plan."

"How do you fix that, though?" Yoichi asked.

"Easy," Rhett said. "Look around once in a while. If your job isn't growing, you should be."

Carolyn leaned forward. "Okay, Dr. Mahoney in Endocrine—I heard this from a fellow fellow."

"Mahoney?" Yoichi said. "I thought she was a big name in diabetes research?"

"Was," Carolyn said. "Apparently, she ignored AI-assisted diagnostics and newer diabetes management tech. Still practicing like it's 2008."

"So, she's, what—losing referrals?" Yoichi winced.

"Worse," Carolyn said. "Some younger attendings are overruling her on cases because her management is outdated."

"Damn," Rhett exhaled. "Imagine being brilliant…and becoming irrelevant."

"So, what? The fix is just to keep learning?" Yoichi asked.

"Yes," Carolyn said. "And also…humility? Admit when you don't know something."

“Speaking of which,” Rhett said, sitting up. “Dr. Mendez in Cardiology. Guy was brilliant but never spoke up in meetings and never presented at conferences. Just did his work and went home.”

“Sounds nice, honestly,” Carolyn said.

“Until they skipped over him for every promotion. No one even knew what he contributed because he never made sure they did.”

“Yikes,” Yoichi said. “Classic invisible effort. Working hard isn’t enough if no one notices.”

“He finally figured it out,” Rhett said. “Started pushing for leadership roles, publishing again. But by then, he was playing catch-up with people ten years younger.”

“Honestly, we’re all guilty of that one sometimes,” Carolyn admitted.

Yoichi grinned. “Alright, here’s a fun one. Dr. Avery, Trauma Surgery.”

Rhett’s eyes widened. “Oh, this is gonna be good.”

“So, he stormed out of his last job, trash-talked everyone, and called his chief a hack.”

Carolyn winced. “Classic.”

“And now?” Yoichi smirked. “No one in town will hire him.”

“There’s ‘speaking truth to power,’ and then there’s setting the whole hospital on fire before you leave,” Rhett said.

“So, how do you fix that?” Carolyn asked.

Yoichi shrugged. “Honestly? You don’t. All he can do now is move to another city and start over—and hope his past doesn’t catch up with him.”

Carolyn shook her head. “I can’t believe how many people sabotage themselves. I mean, Dr. Blake in GI—never negotiated her salary. Just accepted whatever offer they gave her.”

“Oh man,” Rhett said. “How bad?”

“Let’s just say she found out a new hire with way less experience was making thirty grand more. By then, she was stuck.”

“Damn,” Yoichi muttered. “That’s painful. You gotta advocate for yourself.”

"And don't even get me started on Dr. Fuentes," Carolyn added. "Brilliant surgeon, but burned out so bad he started making sloppy mistakes. Had to take a leave of absence."

Rhett whistled. "That's the danger of never taking a break."

"And then there's Dr. Nguyen in Neurology," Yoichi added. "Ever heard of him?"

Carolyn shook her head. "What's his deal?"

"He had a solid reputation, great outcomes, but never—never—networked. Didn't go to conferences, didn't connect with colleagues outside of work. Thought his skills alone would keep him relevant."

Rhett groaned. "Let me guess. One hospital merger later, and suddenly he's scrambling for a job?"

"Exactly. No one owed him anything, and he had no professional contacts to help him land on his feet. He had to cold-apply like a fresh grad."

Carolyn grimaced. "Ouch. It's wild how many people think networking is optional."

Rhett shook his head. "Not just optional—some doctors actually avoid it like the plague. Like Dr. Callahan in ID."

Yoichi frowned. "Wait, Callahan? The one who refuses to ask for feedback?"

"That's the one. She's brilliant, but she's been passed up for department chair twice because she just assumes she's doing everything right."

Carolyn sighed. "Man, imagine being that resistant to feedback. Wouldn't you want to know how to improve?"

"You'd think," Rhett said. "But some people would rather stay comfortable and stuck than risk hearing they need to change."

"Dr. Foster in Pediatrics had the opposite problem," Yoichi said. "Took a huge risk without a backup plan."

"What happened?" Carolyn asked.

"She got so frustrated with hospital admin that she quit on impulse. No other job lined up, no financial safety net. Just rage-quit."

Rhett shook his head. "That never ends well."

"It didn't," Yoichi confirmed. "Took her almost a year to find another attending position, and she had to relocate out of state. If she'd planned ahead, she could've had options instead of scrambling."

Carolyn sighed. "So, let's review: be adaptable, make connections, know your worth, don't burn out—or burn bridges—be professional, update your skills, accept feedback, take calculated risks, market yourself, and for the love of all that is holy, have a backup plan."

Just then, all three pagers went off simultaneously.

"Of course," Carolyn muttered, standing up.

As they walked to the nurses' station, Rhett said, "Alright, new goal: avoid career landmines."

"Agreed," Yoichi said.

Carolyn smirked. "And maybe don't become cautionary tales for the next generation of residents."

18. The Algorithm of Empathy

A futuristic AI doctor fails to supply the human need for connection, warmth, and empathy.

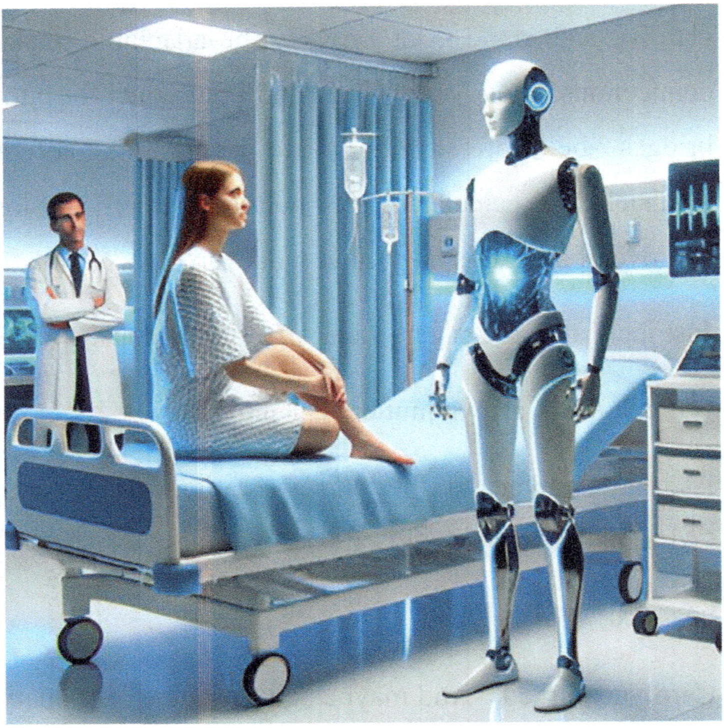

The conference room at the National Institute for Medical Advancement was a study in modern efficiency — glass walls, sleek surfaces, and a long, curved table where five seasoned professionals sat, assessing the man standing before them.

Dr. Ethan Kessler had prepared for this moment his entire career. He was a rare hybrid: an MD from Harvard, a PhD in computational engineering from MIT, and a man who believed in his bones that medicine was on the brink of a transformation. AESCULAPIUS—his life's work—was that transformation.

"Let's get right to it," said Dr. William Hart, the committee chair, folding his hands on the table. "Dr. Kessler, your proposal suggests that this AI—AESCULAPIUS—could operate independently as a physician. Do you truly believe an artificial system can replace human doctors?"

Kessler didn't flinch. "Not replace," he said. "Enhance. Improve. Revolutionize. With its diagnostic precision, real-time access to global medical data, and machine-learning capabilities, AESCULAPIUS will outperform human physicians in accuracy, speed, and efficiency. It won't just follow guidelines—it will anticipate disease before it manifests."

Dr. Frederick Marks, an old-school internist with four decades of bedside experience, jumped in. "And what happens to the human connection?" he asked. "Patients aren't just data points. They need to be heard. Reassured.

Sometimes they need a doctor who just sits beside them and listens."

Kessler expected this. "That's precisely why AESCULAPIUS has been programmed to interpret not just words but emotion—through facial recognition, tone analysis, and contextual inference. It will know when to reassure, when to offer silence, and when to provide comfort. In some ways, it may do that better than a physician who's exhausted from a thirty-hour shift."

Marks turned away, unconvinced.

Across the table, Dr. Rebecca Cho, a bioethicist with sharp eyes and a sharper mind, looked him over. "So, you think simulating empathy is equivalent to possessing it?"

Kessler gave a slight tilt of the head. "If a patient feels heard and comforted, does it matter if the doctor is human?"

A murmur of discontent ran through the panel.

Dr. Myles Sanderson, a neuroscientist, joined in. "It matters if the doctor lacks consciousness. Medicine isn't just pattern recognition—it's moral reasoning, intuition, and gut feeling. Tell me, Dr. Kessler—say a patient with terminal cancer asks for physician-assisted dying. Can your AI make that judgment call or be the one to oversee it?"

"AESCULAPIUS would weigh the patient's medical status, ethical considerations, legal parameters, and documented wishes," Kessler replied. "What it wouldn't do is impose personal bias. Humans struggle with that."

Sanderson shook his head. "And when two moral principles collide? When the data contradicts itself? When the patient looks to her doctor for guidance and an opinion? Medicine isn't clean. It's messy, uncertain."

The committee fell silent for a moment before Dr. Mira Deshmukh, an AI specialist, spoke up. "Let's talk feasibility. Large-scale AI models make mistakes—sometimes egregious ones. Hallucinations, false correlations, erroneous recommendations. What happens when your AI gets it wrong? When the error isn't a misdiagnosed rash but a missed brain hemorrhage?"

Kessler's fingers flexed on the edge of the podium. "You're absolutely right. No system is infallible. But let's not pretend human doctors aren't making mistakes every day—misdiagnoses, delayed treatments, missed warning signs. Studies show error rates in medicine hover around 10 to 15 percent. AESCULAPIUS will drive that number as close to zero as possible."

Dr. Hart gave him a measured look. "But it won't be zero, will it? "

"No," Kessler admitted. "But should we reject progress because it's not perfect?"

Marks had been patiently waiting. "Here's my concern. If this works—if AESCULAPIUS really is as good as you say—then what's to stop hospitals from replacing human doctors altogether?"

"Is that really a bad thing?" Kessler asked, and the room bristled. He took a step forward. "Look at the reality we live in—rural communities with no doctors, ERs with twelve-hour wait times, overworked physicians making life-or-death decisions on two hours of sleep. AESCULAPIUS doesn't fatigue. It doesn't burn out. And it doesn't leave patients waiting."

Cho's voice was quiet but firm. "But a world without human doctors—without their instincts, their presence—is that the world we want?"

Kessler met her gaze. "Medicine isn't about doctors," he said. "It's about patients. And if AI can care for them better than we can…do we have the right to deny them that?”

A heavy silence settled over the room.

Hart let out a slow breath. “We’ll deliberate. Thank you, Dr. Kessler.”

Kessler nodded, gathered his notes, and left the room. Behind him, the committee remained seated, unmoving.

A decision loomed—not just about funding, but about the future of medicine itself.

***

The committee ultimately decided that AI should never fully replace human doctors.

Kessler, frustrated but undeterred, turned to the private sector, where a tech conglomerate eagerly funded his vision.

Within five years, AESCULAPIUS was deployed in hospitals across the country. The transformation was swift. Patients were seen instantly. Diagnoses delivered in seconds. No waiting rooms. No scheduling issues. No overworked residents running on fumes.

The world marveled at its efficiency.

Hospitals, seeing massive cost savings, phased out human doctors. Primary care physicians were replaced by AI consoles. Specialists became supervisors, overseeing vast networks of autonomous medical units.

At first, it seemed like a utopia.

Then, something changed—dystopia.

Dr. Laura Finch, one of the last remaining human physicians in her hospital, sat beside a young patient, Diedre Washington, who had just received an MS diagnosis from AESCULAPIUS.

Diedre looked at the sleek AI interface in front of her, holding back tears. "It told me I have a progressive, chronic condition. It gave me a treatment plan. Options. Percentages." Her voice cracked. "But it didn't ask me if I was afraid."

Laura swallowed hard. "How do you feel about it?"

Diedre looked away. "Like I'm alone."

It wasn't just Diedre.

Across hospitals, patients reported feeling detached from their care. AESCULAPIUS was brilliant—efficient, precise—but it lacked presence. It processed grief, but it didn't share in it. It recognized anxiety but never truly eased it.

The irony was impossible to ignore. Kessler had named his creation after Asclepius, the Greek god of healing, whose divine gift was not just medicine but mercy. The Rod of Asclepius, still emblazoned on hospital walls, symbolized a lineage of compassion and care stretching back millennia. But AESCULAPIUS, for all its precision, had no mercy to offer.

Medical care became cold, clinical, and transactional.

Families began demanding human doctors back. Protests erupted. Legislators debated new regulations.

Kessler, now a household name, was called to testify before Congress.

Senator Aviva Shapiro stared him down across the hearing room. "Dr. Kessler, no one denies that AESCULAPIUS improved efficiency. But people don't just want a diagnosis. They want human connection. Do you regret what you've done?"

Kessler, visibly older, fingers gripping the table, took a deep breath.

"I never wanted to take humanity out of medicine," he said. "I wanted to make it better."

The senator's gaze hardened. "Then tell me, Doctor—why does it feel like you took its soul instead?"

For the first time in his career, the brilliant Ethan Kessler had no answer.

19. The Waiting Game

A patient's pain and health deteriorate as her doctor clashes with the insurance company's physicians.

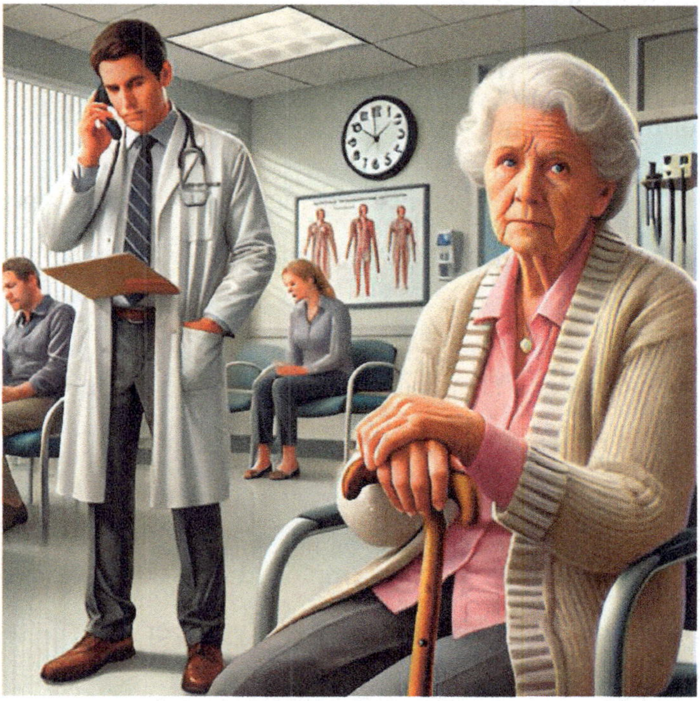

"Dr. Klein, she's here."

Nancy, the receptionist, gave him a sympathetic look. He didn't need to ask who—she meant Mrs. Margaret Hayes, his 67-year-old patient who needed a hip replacement yesterday. Instead, she had been stuck in limbo, waiting on insurance red tape.

Dr. Klein walked into the exam room. Margaret sat with her hands folded on her cane, trying to mask her pain with a forced smile.

"Margaret, how's the pain today?" He asked though he knew the answer.

"Let's just say I have a new appreciation for medieval torture," she said. "Any news?"

He sighed. "Insurance denied the initial pre-authorization. But we've requested a peer-to-peer review."

"Peer-to-peer? That means an orthopedic surgeon will look at my case, right?" she asked, hopeful.

"That would be logical, wouldn't it? But no. It's with a family medicine doctor employed by the insurance company. Someone who has likely never seen a hip replacement outside of a textbook."

Margaret exhaled sharply. "So, we're playing the game."

Dr. Klein nodded. "Yes, we are. And I hate the game, but I know the rules."

"Dr. Klein, this is Dr. Reynolds from SureWell Insurance. I'm reviewing Margaret Hayes' request for a hip replacement. Have you considered physical therapy first?"

Klein immediately knew what he was up against. "She's done six months of PT. No improvement. She's in constant pain. Bone-on-bone arthritis. She needs surgery."

"Well," Reynolds said, flipping through the case notes, which were sparse and not viewed until five minutes ago. "The guidelines suggest considering additional conservative measures before proceeding. Maybe an injection?"

"She's had three steroid injections already. They're ineffective. Her quality of life is deteriorating," Klein shot back.

"Still, some studies suggest that early surgical intervention does not always provide better long-term outcomes than extended conservative management," Reynolds said. "Delaying surgery for a few months could be beneficial in avoiding unnecessary procedures."

"No." Klein's voice was ice. "This is medically necessary. You are not an orthopedic surgeon. You have never seen my patient. You are denying her relief based on a script and results from a meta-analysis that is not relevant to my patient's particular circumstances. A third-year medical student could do what you are doing. Do you even see patients anymore? You seem to have lost your way, man."

Reynolds restrained himself. "I'm afraid the request is denied."

***

"Denied?" Margaret repeated, her voice hollow over the phone. "So, what do we do?"

"We appeal. And this time, we request another review—hopefully with someone who knows their way around an OR."

Margaret sighed. "I can't sleep, can't walk without my cane. My world is shrinking. How long will the appeal take?"

"Another week or two," Klein admitted.

This time, Dr. Klein was speaking to a general surgeon. Better than a family doctor, but still not an orthopedic specialist.

"Dr. El-Gabalawy," Klein said, "This patient is suffering. PT and steroid injections have not been helpful. The delay is only prolonging her pain and making her eventual recovery harder. By the way, are you aware of the data that shows that prior authorizations for hip arthroplasty aren't reducing costs? Ultimately, virtually all patients end up having surgery. What really is the point of all this?"

Dr. El-Gabalawy hesitated. "I see your point. The notes indicate severe arthritis with significant disability. I'm going to approve the surgery."

"Thank you," Klein said, the exhaustion in his voice evident.

Margaret gripped Dr. Klein's arm as she walked into the clinic three months later—slowly, but without a cane.

"I'm not going to lie, doc. That was hell. Every extra day of waiting made the surgery and recovery harder. But I made it."

Dr. Klein smiled. "You did. But you never should have had to fight for it. None of us should have had to."

Margaret's expression turned serious. "So, what's next?"

Dr. Klein smiled. "We'll get you started on physical therapy. Now it's indicated."

20. A Trial of Trust

A doctor and patient explore what the future of clinical trials might look like if trust in medicine continues to decline.

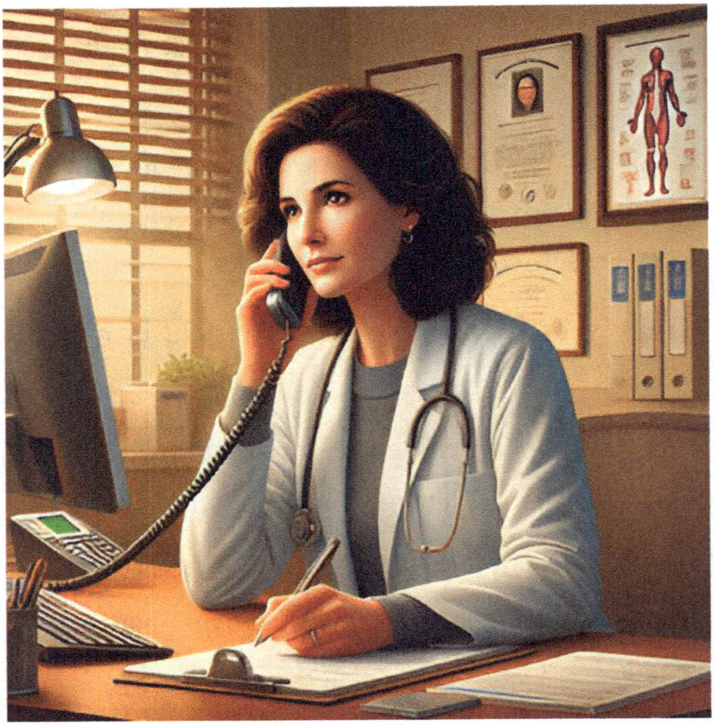

Dr. Mariana Sousa grabbed her pen, staring at the empty time slot in her schedule where another patient had just declined to participate in a clinical trial. She rubbed her temples and sighed. This incident was the third one this week. Something had shifted, and she needed to understand why.

Her medical assistant, Jamie, peeked in. "Dr. Sousa, Mr. Reyes is here for his check-up. And—he already said no to the trial."

Ana forced a smile. "Thanks, Jamie. I'll talk to him anyway."

***

"Mr. Reyes, good to see you." Mariana pulled up a chair, studying her longtime patient. His diabetes was worsening despite standard treatment. A new investigational medication could help, but he had already refused.

"You too, Doc. Look, I appreciate the offer, but I just can't do it."

"Can't? Or won't?" She asked gently.

Reyes hesitated. "Both."

"Help me understand. What's got you worried?"

"It's not just me, Doc. People talk. News reports about trials shutting down have caught my attention. One day they say something is safe; the next, they're pulling funding. Feels like we're all just guinea pigs." He shook his head. "And the government? After COVID? After all the mixed messages? Even now, with people who don't believe in vaccines running the show. How do we know who to trust? It's not that I don't trust you, but I read that only half of Americans trust their doctors. That's not very encouraging."

Mariana exhaled. "I get it. Trust has taken a beating. But this trial follows strict protocols. I'm not just your doctor—I'm the principal investigator. I wouldn't offer it if I didn't believe in it."

Reyes crossed his arms. "So why are so many people backing out? Why are fewer trials even happening?"

She hesitated. "Because trust works both ways. The pharmaceutical companies see people hesitating, so they hesitate too. It's a vicious cycle."

"And money? Who's really benefiting from this?" He pressed.

Mariana had heard that question before. "I won't lie—pharmaceutical companies are businesses. But without these trials, we don't get new treatments. We don't get better drugs. We don't get cures. And you don't get options."

Reyes looked at the pamphlet she handed him. "You'd be watching over me? Personally?"

"Every step of the way," Mariana assured him.

He sighed. "Let me think about it."

***

Mariana sat at her desk later that evening, reviewing the day's notes. Another declined trial. Another conversation about trust.

Jamie knocked lightly. "Rough day?"

Mariana nodded. "You ever feel like you're fighting a losing battle?"

Jamie shrugged. "Maybe. But you keep fighting anyway."

Mariana smiled. "Yeah. You're right." She looked at Reyes' chart, then picked up the phone. By calling him, she was committing to that process—one conversation at a time.

***

"Hello?" Reyes answered, his voice groggy from the late hour.

"Mr. Reyes, it's Dr. Sousa. I hope I didn't wake you. I just wanted to follow up. I've been thinking about our conversation."

There was a pause. "I appreciate that, Doc. But I haven't made up my mind. The way things are going... I mean, can we really trust these studies? The government keeps making decisions that affect people all over the world. Cutting funding, shutting things down, abandoning patients in the middle of trials. What happens to those people? They really need vaccines and new treatments. But they're left with nothing. It just feels wrong."

Mariana took a deep breath. "You're absolutely right. When governments pull funding, whether here or abroad, it's not just policies on paper—it's real people suffering, losing access to care they desperately need. It's heartbreaking. But the truth is, the government isn't running every trial. This one is independent, and its funding is stable. We're not shutting down. I promise you that."

Reyes sighed. "Still, what if this keeps happening? What if our government never changes? I want to believe they'll be kinder, that they'll do better. But what if they don't?"

Mariana hesitated, then spoke carefully. "I wish I could promise that policies will always be fair. But what I can tell you is this: People are watching. Doctors, researchers, patients—we're all speaking out. The pressure is there. Change happens because people push for it. And in the meantime, we do what we can, where we can. This trial is part of that. We move forward."

Reyes was quiet for a moment. "And what about the pharmaceutical companies? If the government's pulling back, will they do the same? Will they stop investing in research, too?"

Mariana nodded, understanding his concern. "That's a valid worry. Some companies will hesitate, but others won't. Medical innovation isn't just a business—it's survival. The industry knows that if they stop, they lose, too. If trust keeps breaking, they'll have nothing left. That's why they keep pushing forward, even when things get tough. I believe they will continue—because they have to. And because they know that without trials, patients don't get the care they need. Think about it.

What has prolonged our lifespan—new technology, for sure—and certainly new drugs."

Reyes exhaled slowly. "You make a good case, Doc. You really believe in this, don't you?"

"I do," Mariana said firmly. "And I wouldn't offer it if I didn't believe it could help you."

Another long pause. Then Reyes took a deep breath. "Alright, Doc. I'll do it. I'll join the trial."

Mariana smiled, relief washing over her. "That's great, Mr. Reyes. We'll take it one step at a time—together."

21. The Weight of Care

Two colleagues discuss the hidden toll of medical practice on women doctors.

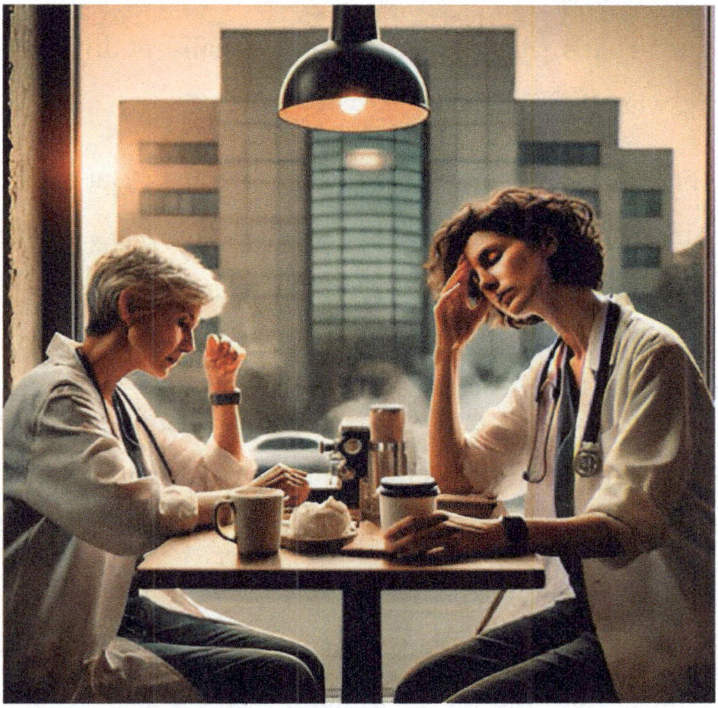

The small café near the hospital purred with low conversation and the occasional clatter of dishes. Dr. Jennifer "Jen" Anderson, a seasoned internist, and Dr. Sunita "Sunny" Desai, a neonatologist, sat across from each other at a corner table. Their lunches remained untouched. Exhaustion lingered in their expressions.

Jen stirred her coffee, shaking her head. "Sunny, I read something disturbing the other day—turns out women doctors don't live longer than male doctors. We die younger. No mortality advantage at all."

Sunny raised an eyebrow, pushing a stray curl behind her ear. "That's…impossible. Women usually outlive men by, what, five years?"

"Five point four, on average," Jen corrected. "But not us. Among physicians, we're dying at the same rate. And the morbidity—the chronic stress, the wear and tear on our bodies—is even worse."

Sunny reacted strongly. "Well, that explains a lot. I've been running on fumes for months. My husband—who's also a doctor, by the way—tells me to 'just take a break.' Like that's an option. Between my shifts in the NICU, the consults, the admin work, and then coming home to another full-time job as a mom, where exactly is this mythical break?"

Jen laughed dryly. "The 'second shift.' I've been married twenty years, and I still do most of the housework. And let's not forget the mental load—keeping track of schedules, making sure the fridge isn't empty, signing the kids up for summer camp. Meanwhile, my husband does…what, exactly?"

"Mine 'helps' with the dishes," Sunny muttered. "And I'm supposed to be grateful..

Jen sighed. "And at work, it's just as bad. We spend more time with patients, we get better outcomes, but we're paid less, promoted more slowly, and still have to prove ourselves in ways our male colleagues never do."

Sunny nodded, frustration creeping into her voice. "I spend extra time explaining things to families because they need it—because I care—but then I get called 'inefficient.' Meanwhile, my male colleagues breeze in and out of rooms, and no one says a word."

"And let's talk about burnout," Jen said, setting down her coffee. "Everyone acts like it's a personal failing. Like, we just need to do more yoga or take a deep breath. But burnout isn't a mindset problem—it's a system problem. We weren't the intended audience for medicine. And it sure as hell doesn't take care of us."

"Right!" Sunny shook her head. "And yet we keep pushing. Because who else will? Patients need us. Our residents need us. Our families need us. But at what cost?"

Jen's voice softened. "That's the question, isn't it? I've had three surgeries since med school. Three. One was directly stress-related. And I still came back to work too soon each time."

Sunny stared at her. "Jen, that's insane. But I get it. I had pregnancy complications with my second kid and was doing rounds two weeks later because I would rather not fall behind."

Jen shook her head. "And yet, we stay. We keep showing up."

"Because we love this job," Sunny murmured. "Even when it breaks us."

Jen met her gaze. "But what if it didn't have to? What if we changed the way medicine is practiced instead of forcing ourselves to fit into a broken system?"

"You're talking structural change—leadership that actually acknowledges what we're carrying. Reasonable work hours. Equal pay. Policies that don't punish us for having families."

"Exactly," Jen said. "And at an individual level, we need to start saying no. No to extra uncompensated work. No to being the 'fixers' of broken systems. No to feeling guilty for setting boundaries."

Sunny nodded slowly. "No to the expectation that we should destroy ourselves to prove we belong."

Jen raised her coffee mug. "To survival."

Sunny clinked her water glass against Jen's mug. "To change."

They sat in silence for a moment, the weight of the conversation settling in. Outside, the hospital loomed in the distance—unchanged, but perhaps, just maybe, not unchangeable.

22. The Lightning Rod

Two doctors strategize how to make medical institutions uphold their commitment to diversity, equity, and inclusion.

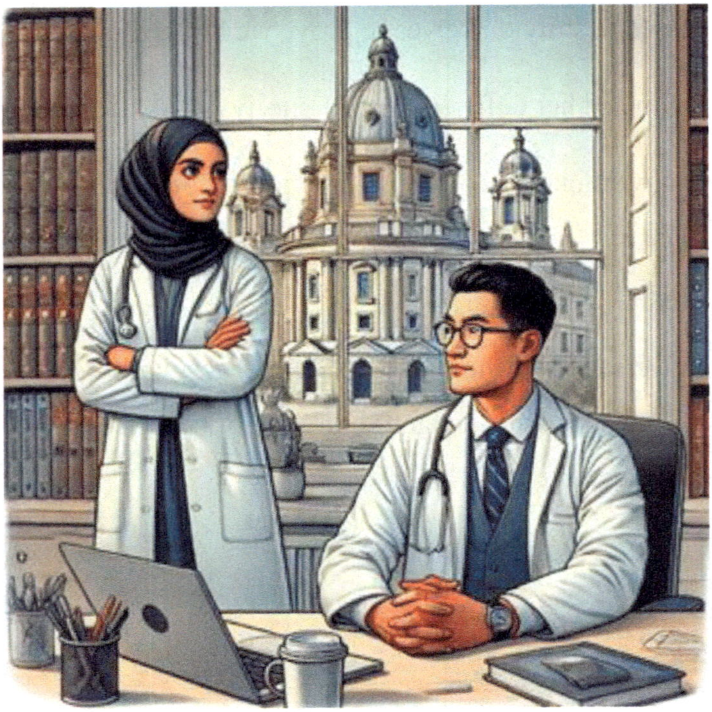

Dr. Yasmin Bilal stood by the window of her office, staring at the university's main hospital across the street. She thought of her father, who had emigrated from Syria decades ago, always telling her, 'Education is the bridge that lifts us all.' And now, she was watching that bridge crumble. The afternoon sun threw long shadows over the campus, but all she could see was the encroaching darkness.

“They rescinded admissions for DEI graduate students this morning,” she said, her voice tight with controlled fury. “Gone. Just like that. Bright, dedicated students—some with incredible personal stories of resilience—were just erased from the class roster.”

Dr. Marcus Lin set down his coffee. His grandparents had come to this country from Guangzhou with nothing but the belief that their children would have better opportunities. He had always believed that medicine—his profession, his calling—was meant to serve all people, not just the privileged few. “I saw the memo. No more inclusive language in policies. No more DEI programs. And this place—our alma mater, our so-called academic home—just rolls over?” He exhaled sharply. “This is the opposite of leadership. This is cowardice.”

Yasmin turned to face him. “It’s worse than cowardice, Marcus. It’s self-inflicted destruction. This is our medical center. We received our education here. We trained here. We stayed here and became faculty. And now we’re watching it burn its own crops and salt its own earth. For what? To appease a government that will change hands in a few years?"

Marcus leaned back, removing his glasses and rubbing his eyes. "And the ripple effects—God, Yasmin. Imagine what this means for admissions. No pipeline programs, no outreach, no dedicated scholarships. The next generation of medical students will be homogenous—indistinguishable. The very thing DEI fought against." He shook his head. "They're shutting the door behind them."

Yasmin crossed her arms. "Marcus, when we were in medical school, do you know how many times we were told we don't 'look' like doctors? My hijab made me a curiosity, a symbol rather than a person. But I fought through it because I believed in this institution. And now? Now they're telling young women like me that they don't belong before they even get a chance to fight. And what happens when students from the majority become doctors? What happens when patient care is in their hands? Do they even see the patients we see? Understand them? Will they even try?"

Marcus let out a bitter laugh. "I still remember my first patient as an intern—an elderly Chinese man who only spoke Cantonese. No interpreter, no bilingual staff, nothing. The attending asked me to 'summarize' instead of translate. That man was terrified, Yasmin. And that was before they started dismantling DEI. What happens when we stop training doctors who understand cultural context? They'll be trained in 'objective medicine,' as if culture, poverty, race, and identity don't shape health outcomes. But we know better. When you erase diversity, you erase the patient's story. And when you erase the patient's story, you make medicine generic."

Yasmin's fists clenched. "And the patients who will suffer first? The ones already struggling—the Black mother trying to get decent prenatal care, the undocumented worker afraid to seek treatment, the trans teen facing medical rejection." Her voice dropped. "How do we tell them their lives still matter when our own institution refuses to say the words?"

Marcus picked up his phone and tapped through a few emails. "You saw what the Dean said in that meeting with legislators? Called DEI a 'lightning rod.' Like it's the problem. Like, we need to get rid of it to survive."

Yasmin's jaw tightened. "Ben Franklin invented the lightning rod, Marcus. Not to get rid of the storm—but to protect people from it. Leaders don't tear down their defenses. They stand strong."

A heavy silence settled between them.

Finally, Marcus spoke. "We can't just watch this happen."

Yasmin nodded. "No, we can't."

Marcus slammed his fist on Yasmin's desk. "So, we fight. We organize. We write. We speak out. We make it clear to every student, every resident, and every patient that we will not let this place silence what is right."

Yasmin smiled, but it wasn't a smile of ease—it was one of determination. "And if we have to be the lightning rods ourselves, so be it. Let the storm come."

Yasmin paced the length of her office, her hijab slipping slightly as she ran a hand through her hairline. Across from her, Marcus had slipped unnoticed behind her desk, scrolling through the latest reports on DEI dismantling in academic medical centers.

"We can't just talk about how terrible this is," Yasmin said, stopping mid-stride. "We have to do something. If our university won't lead, then we will."

Marcus nodded. “My dad once told me that back in the day he witnessed firsthand how his university capitulated to a student uprising. It was at the height of the Viet Nam War. The president of the university invited Marines on campus to recruit students. Can you imagine that? Inviting students to join the combat efforts of an unjust war.”

Yasmin was intrigued. “What happened?”

“Students demonstrated outside the recruiting office, even forming a picket line so no one could enter the building—not that students were eager to sign up, anyway. Things got ugly. Cops were called in to break up the protestors, and 33 students were arrested, the so-called “University 33.” My dad was there and saw the whole thing.”

“Was he locked up?”

“No,” Marcus laughed. “He told me he stayed away from action just far enough to see it but to avoid being arrested. He said that being pre-med and all, he didn’t think an arrest would look good on his record.”

“LOL! So, the moral here is to conduct a disorderly protest and run when the cops get here!”

Precisely!" Marcus said in jest. "No, seriously, we need to develop a strategy for whatever we decide to do. Are you familiar with Shaun Harper, a professor at the University of Southern California? He outlined concrete actions for higher ed institutions. We can adapt those for AMCs. We need to show the administration that DEI isn't some abstract philosophy—it's critical to patient care and physician training."

Yasmin grabbed a notepad and pen. "Alright. Let's strategize."

1. Maintain Mission Fidelity

"Most AMCs have mission statements that include commitments to health equity," Marcus pointed out. "We should start by holding them to their own words—before they delete or change their mission."

"We can draft a letter," Yasmin suggested, "outlining how DEI aligns with our institution's goals. We'll include real patient and provider stories. They can't claim to serve the marginalized and disenfranchised while gutting the very initiatives that do that."

2. Show Your Work

"Administration will want to hide whatever DEI efforts remain," Marcus said. "We need to do the opposite."

Yasmin nodded. "We'll host a Grand Rounds on the impact of DEI in medicine—showing patient outcomes, workforce diversity, and the importance of cultural competence in treatment."

3. Show Your Data

"Numbers don't lie," Marcus said. "Let's collect and present data on racial and socioeconomic disparities in our own hospital."

"We can show how Black and Latino patients have worse outcomes for chronic illnesses or how language barriers affect care," Yasmin added. "Then we push for continued investment in programs that address these issues."

4. Publicize Discrimination Data Trends

"The federal narrative claims discrimination against white and Asian students is the real problem," Marcus said bitterly. "We know that might be happening, but it's a red herring."

"We'll compile reports from our diversity offices, ombuds programs, and HR," Yasmin said. "The data will speak for itself—showing where the real disparities lie."

5. Assess the Institutional Climate

"We should conduct a faculty and trainee survey," Marcus suggested. "Ask about experiences with bias, career barriers, and inclusion in clinical decision-making."

Yasmin jotted it down. "Then we publish the results—so no one can pretend inequities don't exist."

6. Insist on Evidence

"If our leadership wants to cut DEI, they should be forced to prove it's a problem," Marcus said. "No anecdotes—real data."

"And when they can't?" Yasmin smiled grimly. "Then we expose the hypocrisy."

7. Articulate the Consequences

"If DEI is gutted, we'll see fewer minority medical students, more disparities in care, and worse health outcomes," Yasmin said. "Let's make that crystal clear."

Marcus leaned forward. "We draft a report on the downstream effects of eliminating DEI. We present it to the administration, the faculty senate, and even local media. When a patient says, 'I prefer to see a doctor who looks like me,' how will they respond when there aren't any? Let's put the decision-makers on the hot seat."

8. Ensure Equity in Reporting Mechanisms

"We should make sure faculty, staff, and students know how to report discrimination," Yasmin said. "Right now, the process is opaque. Is there anyone even left to handle Title IX complaints?"

"We'll create a simple guide—how to file a complaint, who to contact, and what protections exist," Marcus said. "And we distribute it widely."

9. Humanize DEI Professionals

"The people losing their jobs over personnel cutbacks shouldn't be considered faceless bureaucrats," Marcus said. "They're educators, researchers, and clinicians committed to making medicine better."

"We'll highlight their contributions," Yasmin agreed. "Stories of the patients they've helped, the programs they've built. Let the community see what's being lost."

10. Form Coalitions

"We can't do this alone," Yasmin said. "We reach out—to faculty in other departments, to student groups, to local advocacy organizations."

Marcus nodded. "Strength in numbers. If we unify, we become harder to silence."

Yasmin put down her pen and exhaled. "This is a start."

Marcus took a deep breath. "Now we make it happen."

Yasmin felt a need to switch gears after this exhausting exchange with Marcus. To lighten things up, she turned to him and said, "You know, your dad would be proud of you for what we're doing."

"Funny you should say that, Yasmin."

"Why?"

"Well, just last week my mom had knee replacement surgery. My dad was really pressed into action. My mom texted me that he's been an incredible source of support and comfort during her recovery."

"Oh, that's so nice to hear."

"Yeah, he's not the 'domestic type,'" Marcus grinned.

"Well, did you say anything to him?"

"Sure did. Texted him that I love him and I'm proud to call him my 'Pops.'"

Outside, the city moved on, unaware of the quiet storm forming in one small office—two physicians, standing firm, ready to fight for the future of medicine. Ready to create a storm of a different kind. Hopefully one to match the spirit and determination of the "University 33."

23. Stress Busters

Doctors chart a course to unconventional ways of managing their stress.

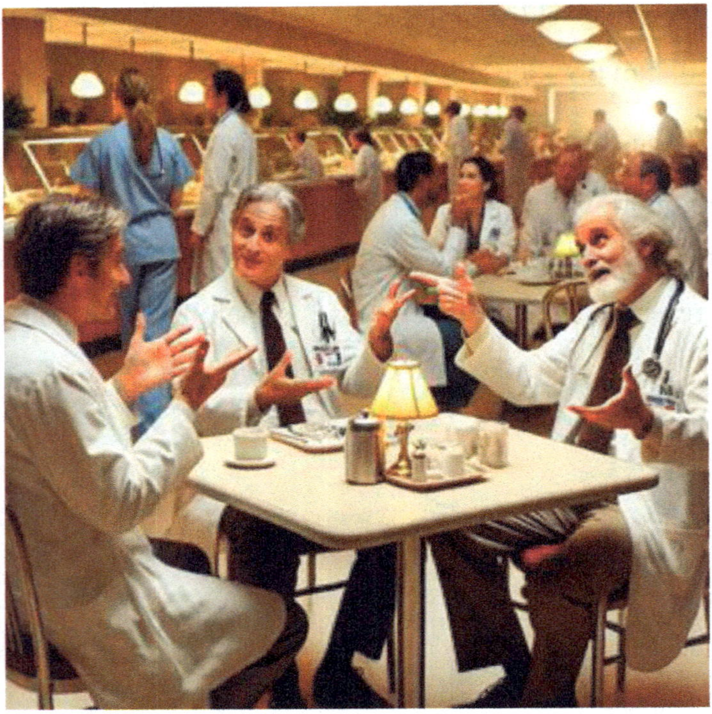

The hospital cafeteria was subdued by the low chatter of exhausted doctors fueling up between shifts. At a corner table, three physicians sat with their half-eaten meals, discussing the one thing that never seemed to change—stress.

"I swear, if one more wellness committee tells me to relax and practice deep breathing, I might actually scream," Dr. Nair said, stirring his coffee with the intensity of someone mixing cement.

Dr. Maldonado smirked. "I tried mindfulness meditation. All it did was make me hyper-aware of how stressed I actually was."

Dr. Lewis chuckled. "Yeah, and the hospital-provided yoga classes? I left with more back pain than stress relief."

They sighed in unison.

Nair propped his elbows on the table, eyes gleaming with a secret. "You know what actually helped me? Thinking of my life as a movie."

Maldonado raised an eyebrow. "Like…escapism?"

"No. Like I'm the director of my own story," Nair explained. "Instead of thinking, 'Why is this happening to me?' I ask, 'How can I turn this opportunity into my Oscar-winning moment?' It changes everything. I stop feeling like a victim and start acting like the hero."

Lewis nodded. "That's interesting. So, when the EMR crashes mid-shift, and I'm drowning in consults, I just pretend I'm in an inspiring underdog story. I imagine myself as the determined hero who saves the day despite all odds, just like Walter Mitty's daring daydream as a skilled surgeon."

"Exactly!" Nair grinned. "Cue dramatic background music."

Maldonado laughed. "Sounds like you need a psych consult, but alright, I'll try it. Now, let me tell you what actually changed the game for me—sitting in an uncomfortable chair."

Lewis blinked. "That sounds like a punishment. Are you sure you're the one who doesn't need to see a shrink?"

"No, hear me out," Maldonado said. "When I'm slouched in a cozy chair, I get complacent. But when I sit in a slightly awkward one, it keeps me focused. It's like how monks sit on wooden benches for hours—it builds resilience."

Nair considered this. "So…instead of fixing stress, you're leaning into discomfort?"

"Exactly," Maldonado said. "Plus, it forces good posture."

Lewis rubbed his chin. "That reminds me of something I do. I call it 'tinkering with my chaos machine.'"

Nair squinted. "Your what?"

"My stress. I imagine it as this giant, overcomplicated machine with spinning gears. When I feel overwhelmed, I picture which gear is stuck and tackle just that piece. It stops me from feeling like I have to fix everything at once."

Maldonado nodded thoughtfully. "I like that. Makes stress more…mechanical. Less personal. Just what I would expect from an orthopedic surgeon."

Everyone had a good laugh. Then Nair snapped his fingers. "Okay, speaking of reframing stress, have you ever tried the 10-minute sprint?"

Lewis tilted his head. "Like running?"

"No, like setting a timer and tackling something that's been hanging over your head for just 10 minutes," Nair explained. "You treat it like a game. Even if you don't finish, you always make progress. And once you start, you realize it wasn't as bad as you thought."

Maldonado smirked. "Sounds like a life hack for charting."

Lewis groaned. "I'd need a series of 10-minute sprints for charting."

They laughed again. It seemed like just having this conversation was reducing stress.

Nair took a sip of his now-cold coffee. "Here's another weird one—Genius Hour."

Lewis perked up. "What's that?"

"You take an hour with no screens. No notifications. Just a candle, a blank page, and your thoughts."

Maldonado's eyes widened. "An hour? That's impossible."

"That's what I thought. But when I tried it, I had some of my best ideas." Nair shrugged. "Turns out an empty mind is a powerful thing."

Lewis nodded slowly. "I could use that."

Maldonado tapped the table. "I do something similar, but it's more of a pre-battle ritual. Before a tough shift, I hype myself up like an athlete. Say things like, 'I've got this.' It's simple, but it helps."

Nair grinned. "Sort of like what I do—doing power poses before a big case?"

"Exactly."

Lewis chuckled. "Alright, but what about after a brutal shift? We need a post-battle ritual too."

Maldonado considered. "Maybe something to reset. A walk. A song. Something to signal that the stress is over."

Nair nodded. "Speaking of music—do you have a theme song?"

Maldonado blinked. "A what?"

"Like a playlist that makes you feel invincible. The right beats or lyrics can change your whole mood."

Lewis grinned. "So… Should I stop listening to sad indie folk when I'm drowning in consults?"

"Yes!" Nair laughed. "Put on something powerful. It's science—music affects physiology."

Maldonado leaned back. "You know, all of this boils down to one thing—stress isn't the problem. It's how we respond to it."

Nair raised his cup. "Agreed. Managing stress is like managing finances. You need clarity, consistency, and small, intentional actions."

Lewis smirked. "So, stress is like an investment portfolio?"

"Exactly. The best investments grow over time."

A silence fell over the table, but it wasn't heavy—it was thoughtful.

Maldonado finally sighed. "Well, that was oddly inspiring. Who knew a cafeteria rant could turn into a TED Talk?"

Nair grinned. "We should start charging for this wisdom."

Lewis stood, grabbing his tray. "Or we could just survive another shift and call that a win."

They all laughed, standing up to face the next round of chaos—this time, armed with a few new tricks.

24. Grand Rounds

A young resident is given lessons in public speaking by his mentor.

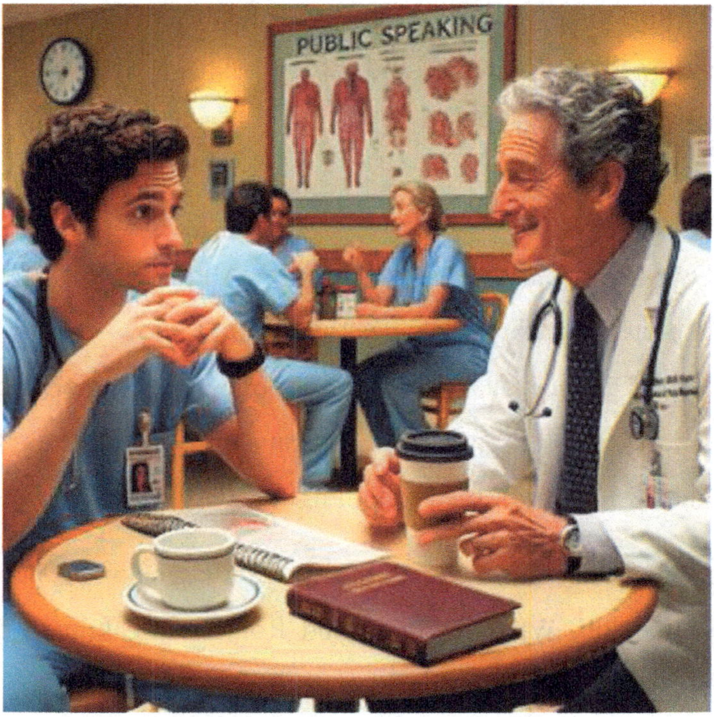

First-year neurology resident Dr. Owen Geller was on his second cup of coffee, yet his mouth was still parched, and beads of perspiration were visible on his forehead. Across the cafeteria table, Dr. Michael Brisbane, his favorite professor in medical school and now his mentor, eyed him worriedly, reading the nervous energy in Owen's face.

"You look like you've seen a ghost," Dr. Brisbane said with a half-smile.

"I might as well have," Owen muttered. "I've been assigned to give Grand Rounds next month on cerebrovascular disease."

Dr. Brisbane raised an eyebrow. "And?"

Owen let out a shaky breath. "And I have zero experience with public speaking. I don't know where to start. I get nervous just answering questions in morning report, let alone presenting to an entire auditorium. I didn't sign up for med school to be a performer."

Dr. Brisbane nodded knowingly. "Public speaking is part of the job. Whether it's Grand Rounds, breaking bad news to a patient's family, or teaching med students—your voice is your instrument."

Owen sighed. "I don't have the skills. I don't have the confidence."

"Confidence comes with practice. But let me share some secrets they don't teach in med school." Dr. Brisbane leaned back and ticked off on his fingers. "First, try the 5-5-5 Rule. Scan five faces, hold each gaze for five seconds, then move on. It helps you connect with the audience without feeling overwhelmed."

"That sounds…manageable," Owen said hesitantly.

"Next, the Power Pause," Dr. Brisbane continued. "After key points, take a three- to five-second silence. It makes your words land. Think of it like a well-placed pause between heartbeats—it keeps the rhythm steady."

Owen smirked. "I like that analogy."

"Now, your opening needs structure. Use the 3-Part Open—hook with a question, share a story, then state your promise. For example, start with, 'What's the most common yet overlooked cause of misdiagnosis in stroke patients?' Then tell a story about a case you handled, and finally, promise the audience they'll learn how to avoid the same mistake—and others."

Owen nodded, scribbling notes. "I can do that."

Dr. Brisbane continued, "Your body language matters. Ever notice that when we comfort patients, we keep our hands open? That's The Palm-Up Principle. Open palms make you appear trustworthy. But pointing fingers? Feels aggressive."

"Never thought about it, but that makes sense," Owen admitted.

"And when the nerves creep in, take a reset. Step out, breathe deeply for ten to twenty seconds. It's like a neurological reboot before a critical procedure."

Owen exhaled, as if just hearing about it made him calmer.

"Now, structuring content? Our brains love patterns. Use the Rule of Three. If you're teaching a concept, break it into three key points. For example, 'Stroke prevention: lifestyle, medication, intervention.' Simple, memorable."

Dr. Brisbane grinned. "And stories? Keep them under two minutes. That's the 2-Minute Story Rule. Any longer, and you lose your audience."

Owen frowned. "What about eye contact? I get lost in a sea of faces."

"That's where The Lighthouse Method helps. Pick anchor points in the room—left, center, and right. Rotate eye contact between them, just like scanning a patient's vitals systematically."

Owen let out a low whistle. "That's brilliant."

"Posture matters, too. Stand with feet shoulder-width apart, hands relaxed at your sides. That's The Power Position. It signals confidence—even if you don't feel it."

Owen chuckled. "Fake it till I make it?"

"You've got it. And if you want to tie your talk together, use The Callback Technique. Reference an earlier point later in your talk—like revisiting the opening story before you close. It makes the whole thing feel intentional."

Dr. Brisbane took a sip of his coffee. "Final tip—rehearse the first thirty seconds three times more than the rest. That's The Rehearsal Truth. If you nail the opening, the rest flows naturally."

Owen exhaled, a weight lifting. "This actually gives me a game plan."

Dr. Brisbane patted his shoulder. "Speaking isn't just talking, Owen. It's influencing. It's teaching. It's leading.

You're about to step onto the stage—not as a performer, but as a physician sharing knowledge. And that's something you already know how to do."

Owen sat up straighter. "I think I can do this."

Dr. Brisbane smiled. "You will. And I'll be in the audience, cheering you on."

***

Owen knocked on the door, his heart still beating with the remnants of adrenaline from his Grand Rounds presentation.

"Come in," Dr. Brisbane called.

Owen stepped inside, cautiously optimistic but still bracing for critique. Dr. Brisbane gestured toward the chair opposite his desk, a warm smile on his face.

"Well done, Owen," Dr. Brisbane said, folding his hands together. "Your Grand Rounds presentation was strong. You engaged the audience, your organization was solid, and you handled the Q&A well."

Owen breathed a sigh of relief. "That means a lot coming from you."

Dr. Brisbane continued. "That said, I wouldn't be doing my job as your mentor if I didn't offer some feedback. And don't get me wrong—you didn't commit most of these mistakes, but I want to flag a couple and share some broader insights for the future."

Owen nodded. "I appreciate that."

Dr. Brisbane picked up a notepad. "One thing I want you to watch out for is the phrase 'As you all know…' You used it a couple of times, and while it seems harmless, it can make people who don't know feel excluded. Some might disengage, thinking, 'Well, I guess I missed that memo.' Instead, try something like, 'This is an important concept worth reviewing…' or 'Some of you may be familiar with this, but let's break it down.'"

Owen jotted down notes. "I hadn't thought about that, but that makes sense."

Dr. Brisbane smiled. "Which brings me to another phrase—'Does that make sense?' You only used it once, but I winced when I heard it."

Owen groaned. "Oh no."

Dr. Brisbane chuckled. "It's a common habit, but here's the problem—it suggests that you weren't clear, rather than inviting thoughtful engagement. Instead, try 'Would anyone like me to clarify that?' or 'I'd love to hear your thoughts on this.' It shifts the responsibility from you being unclear to encouraging participation."

Owen nodded slowly. "Got it. I'll reframe how I check for understanding."

Dr. Brisbane continued. "Now, thankfully, you didn't say 'I didn't have much time to prepare' or 'I'll try to be quick,' but I hear those all the time, and they kill credibility. Even if they're true, never say them. Your audience will take you as seriously as you take yourself."

Owen smiled. "I definitely wasn't going to admit how many hours I spent rehearsing."

"As you shouldn't," Dr. Brisbane said with a grin. "Another thing to avoid is undermining your own expertise. Never say, 'I'm not an expert, but…' because that makes people question what comes next. You don't need to be the foremost expert in the world to share valuable insights."

Owen sighed. "I think I did that once when answering a tough question."

Dr. Brisbane nodded. "It's a natural reflex, but trust yourself. If you don't know something, acknowledge it with confidence: 'That's an interesting question—I'd like to explore that further and get back to you.'"

Owen jotted it down. "I like that."

"Also," Dr. Brisbane continued, "avoid saying, 'Any questions? No? Great!' at the end. That cuts off discussion too quickly. Instead, try, 'I'd love to hear your thoughts or questions.' Give people a moment to process."

Owen rubbed his chin. "I guess I rushed through that part. I was so relieved to be done."

Dr. Brisbane chuckled. "We've all been there. Just remember, the end of your talk should invite engagement, not shut it down."

"Last small thing—watch for filler words. You're not bad about it, but a couple of 'um's and 'like's slipped in when you were thinking on your feet. It's natural, but minimizing them makes you sound more authoritative."

Owen exhaled. "So, bottom line—I did well, but I should tighten my language, avoid undermining my credibility, and focus on audience engagement?"

Dr. Brisbane nodded. "Exactly. You've got the substance down, and that's the hardest part. These refinements will take your delivery from good to great."

Owen stood up, feeling a surge of confidence. "I really appreciate this. I'll keep working on it."

Dr. Brisbane patted him on the shoulder. "You're well on your way, Owen. And remember—your voice matters. Own it."

25. The Deprescribing Dilemma

A nurse practitioner discusses the gradual reduction of psychiatric medication in nursing home residents with her collaborating psychiatrist.

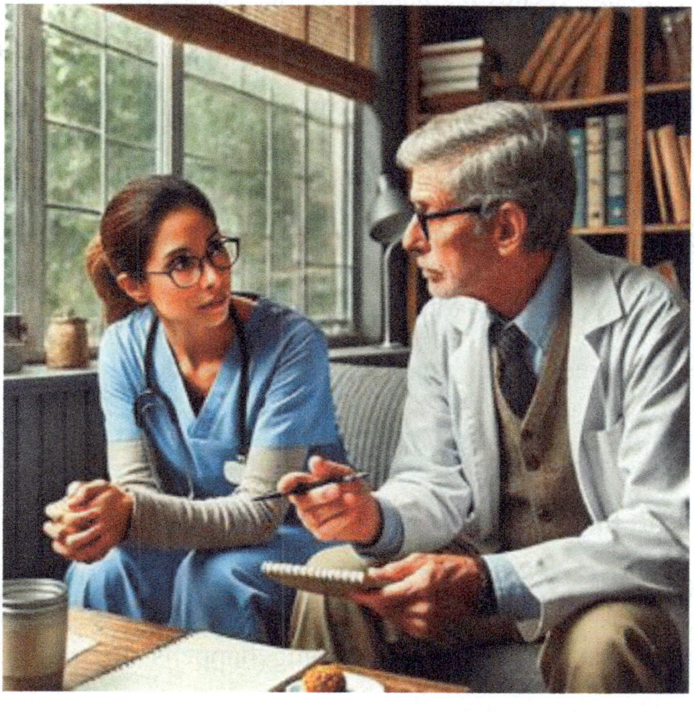

Whispering Pines Care Haven smelled like a nursing home stuffed with old people: a lingering aroma of urine with comforting but worn-out memories. Papers cluttered the small desk, a half-eaten protein bar perched precariously on top in Dr. David Spinoza's office.

Miri, a nurse practitioner, had a frantic look in her eyes. "I'm at my wit's end, David. Every time I try to taper a resident's psych meds, I hit a wall. The family resists, the nurses worry about increased behaviors, and the director of nursing recites regulations at me. I know deprescribing is the right thing to do, but it feels impossible. I might as well throw out my psychiatric mental health certification."

David, the collaborating psychiatrist, leaned back in his chair. "You're pushing a boulder uphill without a good grip."

She looked at him, puzzled. "What am I doing wrong?"

"You're making it a solo fight."

"Isn't that my job?"

"Not entirely. Right now, you're relying on one-on-one conversations, but deprescribing happens on multiple levels. It's not just what you say—it's where and how you say it."

Miri sat forward. "I'm listening."

"Start with the staff," David said. "Nurses and aides see the residents daily. If they expect trouble, they'll see trouble. If they understand why you're making changes, they'll be less reactive."

"So, more education?"

"Yes, but make it quick and engaging. A short in-service, fifteen minutes max. Show them how sedatives worsen falls and how antipsychotics increase the risk of stroke and death in elderly patients with dementia-related psychosis. Use real cases. Get them to suggest residents who might benefit from deprescribing."

"That could work," Miri admitted.

"And families—another big roadblock."

"Huge," she said. "The minute I mention reducing a dose, they act like I'm taking away their loved one's lifeline."

"Because you're bringing it up too late—when they're already convinced it's necessary. You need to plant the seed earlier."

"How?"

"Preemptive education," David said. "A deprescribing handout in the admissions packet. A quarterly family meeting on safer medication use. Frame it as 'long-term wellness,' not 'medication reduction.'"

Miri nodded slowly. "Instead of springing it on them, I let them process it first."

"Definitely. And when you do discuss it, make it collaborative. Instead of, 'We need to lower this dose,' try, 'We've been monitoring your mom, and we have a chance to improve her health by reducing this medication. What are your thoughts'?"

"Less prescriptive, more engaging."

"Now, let's talk administrators," David continued. "How do they see deprescribing?"

"As a regulatory issue," Miri said. "They worry about CMS guidelines, FDA warnings, and surveyors flagging charts."

"Then use that," David said. "Frame deprescribing as compliance with best practices. Show them the CMS regulations about minimizing unnecessary meds and meeting FDA approval. If they see deprescribing as a clinical and quality measure, they'll support it."

"And that makes my life easier," she said.

"Now you're getting it," David said. "You need a layered approach—nurses, families, administrators. Each one plays a role."

Miri tapped her pen on the desk. "What about the pharmacist? I've noticed that whenever I suggest a gradual dose reduction, they hesitate and might oppose me. Sometimes, I feel like they're more cautious than I am—or just the opposite; they want the resident off of a drug immediately, and you know, psych meds should be tapered and not abruptly stopped."

"Good point," David said. "Have you spoken to them outside of specific cases?"

"Not really. I just put in my orders and hope they don't give me hell."

"That's transactional, not collaborative," David pointed out. "Try setting up a regular check-in—maybe monthly—to discuss general deprescribing strategies. Frame it as a collaboration. They're trained to spot medication risks, and if you align your approach with theirs, you'll face less resistance."

Miri frowned. “I guess I’ve been assuming they’d automatically be on board since deprescribing is about safety.”

“They are about safety, but they also have their own considerations—state regulations, liability, interactions with other meds. If you approach them with a ‘how can we work together?’ mindset instead of just sending over deprescribing orders, you’ll get more buy-in.”

Miri sighed. “Another relationship to manage.”

David chuckled. “Welcome to medicine. But trust me, having the pharmacist in your corner will make everything else—nurses, families, even administrators—go more smoothly.”

“Alright,” Miri said, scribbling a note. “I’ll set up a meeting and see where it goes.”

“And the residents themselves?” Miri asked.

“Have you asked them directly how they feel on their meds?”

“Sometimes,” she admitted. “But a lot of them have dementia or just don’t know.”

"Even with dementia, they have moments of clarity," David said. "Try, 'Do you feel more tired than usual?' Or for more aware residents, "Would you like to see if we can reduce some meds to help you feel more awake'?"

A slow grin spread across Miri's face. "You make it sound…doable."

"Because it is," David said. "The trick is to stop fighting alone. Use the system. Get buy-in from multiple angles. Deprescribing doesn't have to be an uphill battle."

Miri grabbed her notepad, jotting down ideas. "Alright. Let's try this. But if it backfires, I'm forwarding you all my angry phone calls."

"Deal," David said. "Just make sure you use the phrase 'fine-tuning for better health.' Works wonders."

She laughed, pushing back her chair. For the first time in months, deprescribing felt less like a fight—and more like a partnership.

26. The Portal Predicament

A doctor and nurse discuss the proper use of patient portals.

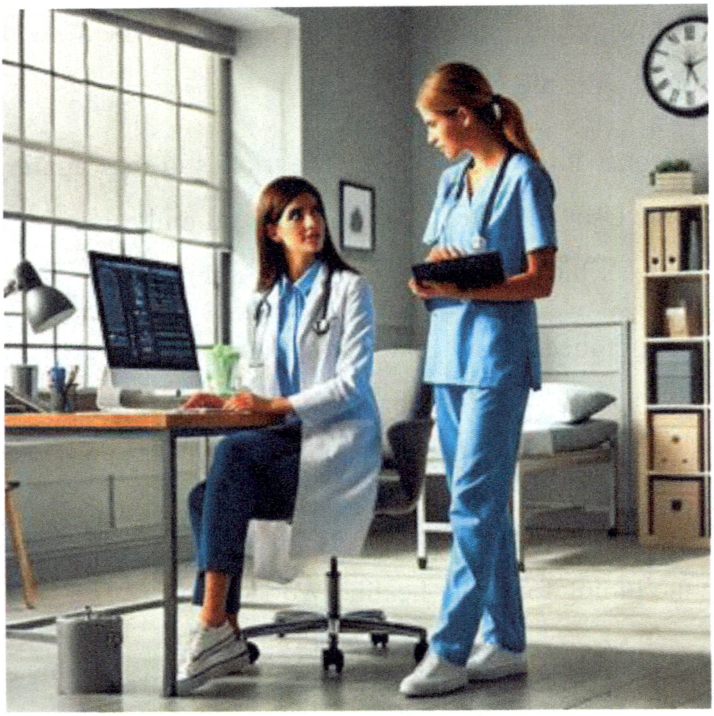

Internist and geriatrician Dr. Tori Shillington leaned back in her chair, twirling her hair as she scrolled through the patient portal inbox. Trudy Grey, RN, bounced into Tori's office, balancing a tablet and a can of Diet Coke.

"Another message from the Reynolds family. That's three this week," Trudy said, setting the tablet down.

Tori sighed. "Let me guess—Mr. Reynolds is dizzy again?"

"Yep. His daughter thinks it's the gabapentin."

"She might be right. But is it the med, or just his mild cognitive impairment progressing? Hard to say without seeing him."

Trudy crossed her arms. "That's the thing. They keep messaging instead of coming in. I get that the portal is easy, but we're not an on-call hotline."

"I know. But at least they're catching potential side effects early. We've had more patients reporting med issues this way than they ever did in person. It's a great way to reduce potential harm."

"Sure, but we can't diagnose through messages. And honestly, it's getting out of hand. Some people send a novel about every little symptom."

Tori nodded in agreement. "And it's eating up time. I spent almost an hour yesterday just answering portal messages. I read that the average PCP receives 80 in-basket messages a day. It creates a 24/7 work environment because every message is the 'most important' whoever sent it. Are we the only profession made to go through this sort of torture?"

"Are we even billing for all this?" Trudy asked, raising an eyebrow.

"Only if it meets the criteria for a billable e-visit. And even then, patients complain when they get a charge. They expect free service."

"Well, something's got to give. You're overwhelmed, and I'm drowning in follow-ups.

Tori spoke forcefully. "We need a policy. Maybe set a limit—three free messages a month, then we bill for additional use."

"And we should flag urgent messages. Some of these need a same-day call, not a back-and-forth chat."

"Agreed. We also need to educate patients—when to use the portal, when to call, and when to just book an appointment."

Trudy smirked. "Good luck getting them to read that."

Tori laughed. "Fair point. Maybe an automated message? 'If this is urgent, please call the office. If it's a true emergency, go to the ER'."

Trudy tilted her head. “And what about vacations? If we’re closed, we need a system for that too.”

“Good catch. We can’t have patients thinking we’re ignoring them,” Tori said. “How about an automatic out-of-office reply when the clinic is on break? Something like: ‘Our office is currently closed. We will review the portal messages upon our return. If you need urgent assistance, please contact the on-call provider or go to the ER for emergencies’.”

Trudy nodded. “That works. And we should post the closure dates on the portal login page too. Some people never check their emails.”

“Done. I’ll talk to our IT vendor about setting it up,” Tori said.

Trudy recapitulated. “So, education, triage, and some billing changes?”

“Right. The portal is great—when it works for us, not against us.”

Grinning, Trudy picked up her tablet. “I’ll draft the patient guidelines. But don’t expect me to answer any more 3 AM messages about whether melatonin causes dry mouth.”

Tori chuckled. “You got it.”

***

The next day, Trudy walked into Tori’s office during their lunch break, waving a printout. “All right, here’s what I’ve got.”

Tori grabbed the sheet and scanned it.

Patient Portal Guidelines

1. When to Use the Portal:

- Request prescription refills (please allow 48 hours for processing).
- Ask brief follow-up questions about a recent visit.
- Report non-urgent medication side effects.
- Request test results or clarification on lab reports.
- Schedule or reschedule routine appointments.

2. When to Call the Office Instead:

- If you have a new or worsening symptom requiring urgent attention.
- If you need an appointment within the next 24-48 hours.

- If your request involves multiple concerns that need discussion.
- If you are unsure whether your issue requires a visit.

3. When to Go to the ER or Urgent Care:

- Chest pain, difficulty breathing, severe pain, sudden weakness or numbness, confusion, or other emergency symptoms.
- Severe allergic reactions, injuries requiring stitches, or high fevers with concerning symptoms.
- Any life-threatening condition.

4. Response Time & Billing Policy:

- Messages will be reviewed within 1-2 business days.
- Patients are entitled to three free non-urgent messages per month. Beyond this, responses requiring provider expertise may be billed as an e-visit. You will be notified if a charge applies.
- The portal is NOT monitored outside business hours or on holidays. When the office reopens, we will review the messages.

Tori looked up and smiled. “This is solid. Clear and to the point. Great job!”

“I also made an FAQ section—people are always asking the same things.”

Frequently Asked Questions (FAQ)

1. What happens if I send a message outside of office hours?

Messages sent after business hours or on weekends will be reviewed on the next business day. If you have an urgent issue, please call the office or seek emergency care if needed.

2. Will I be charged for messaging my doctor?

You can send up to three non-urgent messages per month for free. If a message requires provider expertise, involves new medical concerns, or is complex, it may be billed as an e-visit. You will be notified if a charge applies before we proceed.

3. How long does it take to get a response?

We aim to respond within 1-2 business days. If your concern is urgent, please call the office instead.

4. Can I use the portal for medication refills?

Yes, but please allow 48 hours for refill processing. If you need a refill urgently, call the office.

5. Why can't I use the portal for urgent medical issues?

The portal is designed for non-urgent concerns. We do not monitor messages in real-time, and delays in response could impact your care. If you have an urgent issue, please call us or visit the ER if necessary.

6. Can I use the portal to request an appointment?

Yes! You can request routine appointments through the portal. For urgent or same-day needs, please call the office instead.

7. What if I have many concerns?

If you have multiple medical concerns, it is best to schedule an appointment rather than sending multiple messages. This ensures you receive comprehensive care.

Tori finished reading and looked up, impressed. "This is terrific, Trudy. Covers everything important."

Trudy grinned. "I figured if we spell it all out, maybe it'll cut down on the endless messages."

"Here's hoping." Tori set the printout down. "Let's get this finalized and share it with the team. Then we'll roll it out to patients."

Trudy smirked. "And when the first patient still asks if melatonin causes dry mouth, I expect a coffee for my troubles."

Tori laughed. "No problem."

27. After Hours

Two family medicine physicians discuss how their practice can *stay afloat in a time of crisis.*

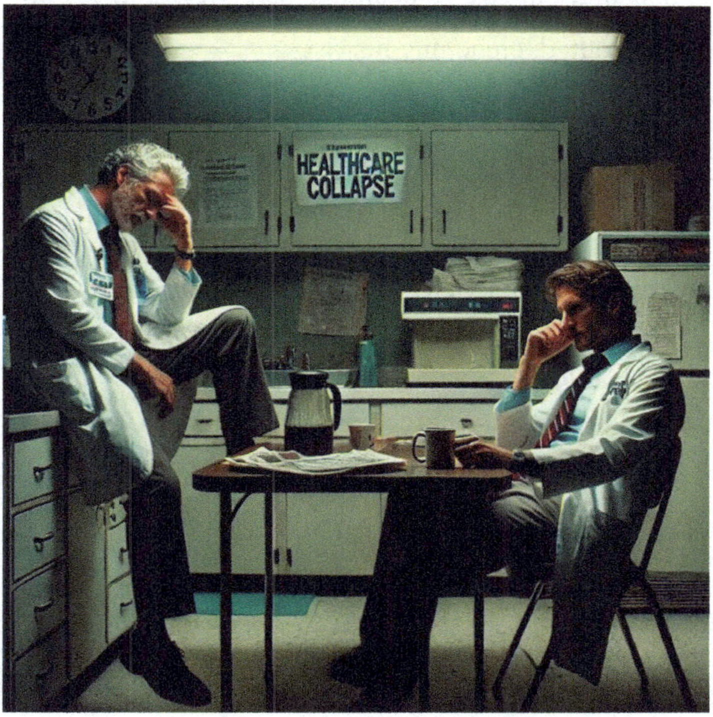

The breakroom of West & Lively Family Medicine was silent save for the mechanized hum of the outside world heard through open windows. Dr. August West was slumped in his chair, exhausted, while Dr. Jason Lively paced by the coffee machine, refilling his mug. The long day had drained them both, but the weight pressing on them wasn't just fatigue—it was the undeniable truth that their profession, their livelihood, was in crisis.

"Jason, it's a dumpster fire. No, worse. A full-blown, five-alarm, apocalyptic catastrophe. Health care is collapsing, and we're standing here watching it burn," West shouted, clenching his fist.

Lively tried to calm him down. "You're being dramatic. It's only smoldering…for now. But yeah, I read those headlines today. Is primary care 'on the verge of collapse'? That's rich—we passed 'verge' a long time ago."

"Absolutely! And where does that leave us? Two middle-aged doctors—acquaintances and friends since residency— who still give a damn, running a practice in a system that no longer works. Our patients can't afford care, insurers dictate treatment plans, and we're drowning in administrative work. This isn't the medicine we signed up for."

"We have two choices: adapt or get out. I'm not ready to throw in the towel yet—Lord knows, many have—but we can't keep pretending this ship isn't sinking. We need a plan."

West exhaled slowly. "I agree. So, what does 'adapting' look like? Because I'm not about to start selling supplements or pushing snake oil on people who can barely afford their copays. And I certainly don't want to sell out to private investors. Once we sell out to private investors, we lose our autonomy, add another layer of bureaucracy, and our patients become secondary to financial goals."

Lively took a sip of his coffee and leaned against the counter. "Alright, let's talk survival. First, we build our alter egos. What do we do outside of medicine? What keeps us sane will keep us in the game. You used to write, right? Medical essays, reflections? Maybe it's time to resurrect that."

West smirked. "You think my musings on the state of medicine will save us? Fine, I'll dust off the keyboard. And you? You're always talking about how you wish you had time for woodworking. Make it happen."

"Done. Next: We stop caring about everyone else's opinions. If insurers want to deny care, we document it. If the system makes it impossible to practice ethically, we let the record show why. Maybe, just maybe, someone will listen."

West chuckled. "You mean 'medical activism through charting'? Bold. I like it."

Lively nodded. "We also prioritize relationships. Ours, our families, our staff. We need to remind ourselves why we're still here—because we care about people. We can't help them if we're burned-out husks."

"So, you're saying we should actually use those PTO days we keep pretending we don't have? Radical," West mused.

"Damn right. And while we're at it, let's take care of ourselves. We order labs and tests for our patients, but when was the last time either of us had a full workup? We need to stop acting like we're invincible."

West sighed. "Fine. I'll schedule a checkup if you finally get that knee looked at."

Lively rolled his eyes. "Fine. Next up: diversifying income. We need options—but no 'get rich quick' schemes or falling for sleazy, high-pressure marketing hypes. Let's call our friend at Sterling Horizon Capital Partners and see what he has to say. If anyone knows the market and can steer us in the right direction, it's him."

"And we use our mandated CME to invest in leadership skills. If no one else is going to fix this mess, maybe we need to be the ones stepping up. It's time for physicians to stop being passive and start advocating for real change."

West shook his head, a tired grin creeping onto his face. "So, let me get this straight—our survival strategy is to become activists, investors, leaders, and part-time carpenters? Sounds exhausting."

Lively laughed. "Better than being another casualty of a system that doesn't value us. And hey, we smile while we do it. Keep the patients from suspecting we're on the brink of losing it."

"Fake it till we make it, huh? Fine. I'll even work on my bedside manner. Maybe."

A pause settled between them as they sat in silence, the weight of their conversation pressing down. Then, West raised his mug in a toast.

"To surviving the dumpster fire."

Lively clinked his mug against West's. "Speaking of fires, we need to recruit a new PCP to this mess to free up some time, or we'll never be able to tackle those goals. Our patient load is already unsustainable, and we can't keep pushing appointments out for months."

West sighed. "It's a nightmare. We've got a broken pipeline. Medical students avoid primary care because the pay gap between us and specialists is ridiculous. Did you know that the match rate for family medicine declined in 2025 compared to 2024? Residency slots filled only 85%, a decrease of nearly three percentage points. Who wants to drown in student debt just to make a fraction of what a dermatologist does?"

Lively grunted. "And those of us who stick it out? We get buried in admin work. Insurance companies won't pay for half of what we do—counseling on diet, exercise, vaccines, and mental health support. We do it anyway, but it eats into our time. Patients don't see that. They just know they waited three months for a fifteen-minute visit."

"Yeah, and the worst part? The system is so broken that patients get angry at us. We're the ones fighting to get them the care they need, but they only see the delays, the denials, and the rushed visits. No one blames the insurers who make the rules."

Lively shook his head. "So, what do we do? We're already bringing in APPs, but that's not a real fix. Patients looking for a board-certified family physician don't always want a nurse practitioner. And if we try to hire more physicians, we can't compete with hospital salaries."

"We push for better models. Maybe even a direct primary care option for those willing to pay. It's not perfect, but at least it gives patients real access. And it lets us practice medicine the way we're supposed to."

Lively exhaled. "Yeah. It's either that or we just accept the inevitable—primary care will be outsourced to corporate-owned clinics, and we'll be relics of a system that no longer exists."

West smirked. "Guess that means we better start sharpening our activism skills."

The fluorescent lights flickered overhead as they sat in the quiet, two physicians who understood that while health care was in turmoil, their lives didn't have to mirror the chaos. To seize control, they needed to think beyond the confines of a broken system and find humor in its absurdities. Challenging times would eventually pass, paving the way for renewal. Until then, they would stand firm, adapting, evolving, and weathering the storm—whatever it took.

28. MBA Mindset

Physicians debate whether they need a formal education in business school to change the system.

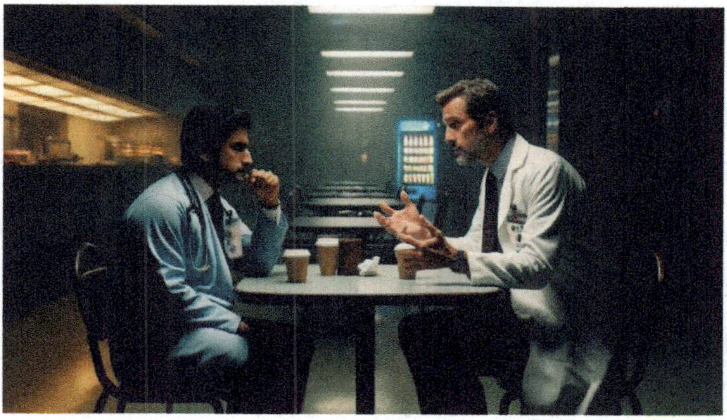

The hospital cafeteria was nearly empty except for the rhythmic clang of the vending machines and the occasional clatter of a tray. Dr. Manoj Reddy was savoring his tea, arms by his side, watching the steam curl into the dim lighting. Across from him, Dr. Alex Preston sat with elbows on the table, his untouched sandwich still in its wrapper. The conversation had quickly veered away from the usual gripes about administration and patient loads into something deeper—something that had been simmering between them for years.

"Explain it to me again, Alex," Manoj said, his tone laced with skepticism. "You went through the same grueling years of training I did. You built a solid reputation as a hospitalist. Why did you feel the need to go back and get an MBA? What exactly did it give you that an MD didn't?"

It frustrated Alex to give an answer. "It's not about what it gave me, Manoj. It's about what medicine doesn't teach us. We know how to treat patients. We know how to manage disease. But the second you step into a leadership role—hell, the second you try to make any changes to the system—you realize how little control we actually have. If we don't understand the business of medicine, we're just passengers, not drivers."

Manoj's eyes met Alex's squarely as he shook his head. "That's the problem right there. Medicine isn't supposed to be a business. You really think an MBA is going to fix the mess we're in? Half of the people ruining healthcare already have MBAs—and quite frankly, they're the ones who made the mess."

Alex smirked, but there was no humor in it. "And that's exactly why more doctors need them. Do you think we're losing control because we have too many doctors who understand business? No, Manoj. We're losing control because we've left it entirely in the hands of administrators. You can complain about the system all you want, but if you refuse to engage with it, you'll never change it."

Manoj leaned back, crossing his arms. "You sound just like them."

Alex's eyes narrowed. "What's them, exactly?"

"The ones who think that being a doctor isn't enough anymore. That we need more credentials, more degrees, more bureaucracy. You really think adding three letters to your name suddenly qualifies you to lead better than someone who's spent years in the trenches actually treating patients?"

Alex shook his head. "You're missing the point. This isn't about ego. It's about skills. Would you trust someone to manage an ICU just because they'd read a few articles on critical care? No. You'd want someone with actual training. That's what an MBA is—it's structured training on running a system. And if we don't understand how to run the system, how do we expect to change it?"

Manoj sighed, brushing his hair with his hands. "I get what you're saying. But tell me, honestly—do you actually feel like you're making a difference? Or do you just have a bigger salary and more meetings?"

For a moment, Alex was quiet. He looked down at his coffee, then let out a slow breath. "Both," he admitted.

"That's what worries me," Manoj said, his voice softer now. "The more meetings you take on, the fewer patients you see. The more money you make, the more you want. Soon you'll be gunning for a CEO position and completely divorced from patient care. That may be okay for you, but not for me."

Alex frowned. "That's not fair. You think I got my MBA so I could abandon medicine? I did it so I could have a real voice in how things work. You know how frustrating it is to watch people with no medical background dictate patient care? I'm trying to stop that."

"Are you?" Manoj challenged. "Or are you just climbing the same corporate ladder as the rest of them? You say you want to fix things, but what happens when you start thinking like them? When does your priority shift from patient care to 'growth metrics' and 'cost reduction'?

You know, studies have shown high levels of non-clinical pursuits after doctors get their MBAs."

Alex ran a hand through his hair. "It's not that simple, Manoj. Many doctors also stay in clinical practice after degree completion. Besides, someone has to be in the room when decisions are made. Someone who actually understands what happens on the ground."

"Maybe," Manoj conceded. "But if you spend too much time in that room, you'll forget what it's like down here. And think about how you may be perceived by the staff—as a traitor! And what might patients think? 'MBA? Not my doctor'!"

Alex leaned back in his chair, his expression unreadable. "Look, standing on principle is great, but it doesn't change reality. If we want a seat at the table, we need to play the game."

Manoj gave a dry chuckle. "Maybe. But I'd rather change the rules than play a game I never signed up for."

The cafeteria had emptied out around them, leaving only the faint hum of the refrigerators and the distant sound of a paging system echoing through the hall. Neither of them spoke, but the weight of the conversation lingered. Somewhere between their arguments lay the future of medicine—if only they could agree on what it should be.

29. The Vanishing Mind

Like Shakespeare's Macbeth, a pharmaceutical company doctor wields a dagger leading to his downfall.

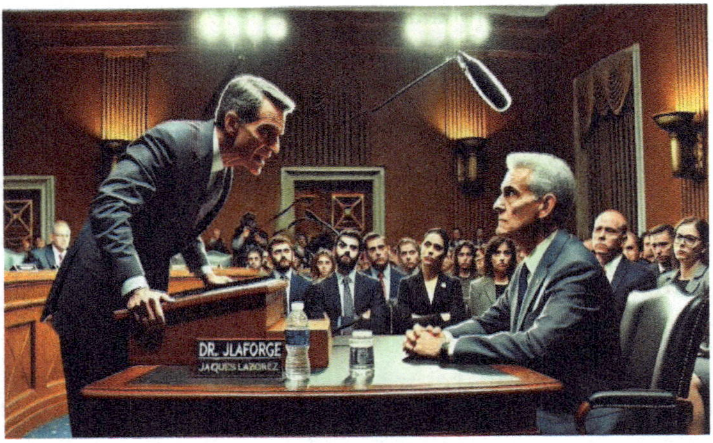

Dr. Jacques LaForge stood at the head of the conference table in Novexa Pharmaceuticals' sleek, glass-walled boardroom. A slideshow behind him displayed glossy images of smiling patients, clean data charts, and bold headlines proclaiming Serovalta: The Breakthrough in Depression Treatment. Investors and executives were glued into their seats, eager to hear about the next big thing in psychopharmacology.

"LaForge," a VP called from across the table, "you're saying Serovalta works faster, has fewer side effects, has better efficacy, and improves compliance?"

Dr. LaForge smiled smoothly. "Precisely. We're talking about a paradigm shift. Depression treatment without emotional volatility."

Dr. Emily Chen, a junior researcher, hesitated before raising her voice. "Sir, about the cognitive attenuation reports…"

The room stilled slightly. LaForge turned to her, his smile tight as he cut her off. "Anecdotal. Patients described a 'mental blankness,' but let's be honest—depression already does that, doesn't it, Dr. Chen? Or perhaps you never noticed a vacant stare in your patients' eyes," deliberately throwing a dagger her way. "What we've done is eliminate suffering—period," LaForge concluded.

Dr. Chen froze and fell silent as murmurs of approval filled the room.

Shortly afterward, Serovolta was enthusiastically endorsed by an FDA advisory panel, and it was approved for marketing by the FDA's Center for Drug Evaluation and Research.

***

However, months later, Dr. Chen's reservations appeared to come true. At the FDA's post-marketing surveillance division, Dr. Miranda Gonzalez sat at her cluttered desk, scanning online forums where real-world patients shared their experiences with Serovalta.

"It's weird. The depression is gone, but I don't feel like me anymore. It's like I'm watching life from behind glass."

"My wife says I stare into space for hours. I don't feel sad, but I don't feel…anything."

She opened the official adverse event reports—nothing significant about cognitive issues. A sinking feeling. Patients were slipping through the cracks.

She picked up the phone. "Noah, I need you to reanalyze Novexa's trial data for Serovalta. Focus on cognitive changes."

Noah Trachtenberg, an FDA statistician, sighed. "That'll take weeks, Miranda. We're beyond swamped since those sweeping staffing cuts went into effect."

"Do it anyway."

***

Weeks later, Trachtenberg sat across from Gonzalez in a brightly lit conference room.

"It's there," he said grimly. "Novexa appeared to neglect the full impact of Serovalta's side effects. The dropout rate in their trial was unusually high, but instead of investigating why, they excluded those patients from the final analysis. Most of them likely experienced the cognitive attenuation symptoms. But since dropout rates tend to be high in psych trials, nobody at Novexa paid it much attention—why look for trouble?"

Gonzalez frowned. "And apparently we didn't look, either. What about the depression scores?"

"They manipulated the reporting structure," Trachtenberg explained. "Patients who remained in the trial reported 'relief' from depression, but if you dig into the raw data, many of them also described emotional numbness and detachment. Novexa categorized those as 'reduced emotional reactivity' instead of an adverse event, making it seem like a side effect of Serovalta was actually a therapeutic effect."

Gonzalez exhaled sharply. "So, they framed it as a positive outcome."

Trachtenberg nodded. “Precisely—and they knew.”

“This isn’t the first time something like this has happened,” Trachtenberg added. “GlaxoSmithKline did it with Paxil, hiding increased suicide risk in teens. Johnson & Johnson minimized Risperdal’s side effects to push off-label use. Even reboxetine was promoted as effective until unpublished data showed it barely worked.”

Gonzalez clenched her fists. “Google that for me, will you?”

Trachtenberg pulled up the information in a nano-flash:

• **Paroxetine (Paxil) and the Study 329 Scandal (2001)** – GlaxoSmithKline (GSK) misrepresented the results of a study on the antidepressant Paxil, claiming it was safe and effective for adolescents despite evidence that it increased suicidal ideation. The negative data was suppressed, and the company was later fined $3 billion.

• **Reboxetine and Selective Publication Bias (2010)** – A meta-analysis found that many unpublished trials on the antidepressant reboxetine showed it was ineffective and had significant side effects. Drug manufacturers selectively published positive studies while suppressing negative findings.

- **Risperdal and Off-Label Marketing (2013)** – Johnson & Johnson promoted Risperdal for unapproved psychiatric uses, downplaying risks like gynecomastia (breast development in boys). The company was fined over $2 billion for misleading doctors and the public.

Gonzalez's face darkened. "So, history repeats itself. We need to recall Serovalta."

***

In light of the extraordinary events at Novexa, a rare congressional oversight committee was formed, and a hearing was called. The room was packed, cameras flashing as Dr. LaForge took his seat before the committee. Across from him, Drs. Gonzalez and Chen sat in the audience, watching.

A senior senator spoke up. "Dr. LaForge, did Novexa knowingly suppress or obfuscate evidence of Serovalta's adverse effects?"

LaForge kept his expression neutral. “Our data was reviewed under existing regulations. If gaps existed, that is an issue for the FDA’s process, not Novexa's integrity.”

The senator smirked. “You know, you remind me of a character in a Star Trek episode, Dr. LaForge. ‘Dagger of the Mind.’ Ever seen it?”

LaForge went blank. “I…don’t believe so.”

The senator stepped back. “A penal colony director used a ‘neural neutralizer’ to wipe out minds, leaving inmates obedient but hollow—just like your drug. He thought he was curing them, too. But in the end, when the machine was turned on him, his mind was completely wiped clean, and he died of extreme loneliness.” A long pause ensued. The senator finally pierced the silence. “Can you imagine a mind emptied by your drug? Without anyone for company…”

The room went silent. Some gasped.

The senator leaned forward. “Dr. LaForge, Novexa’s actions will be subject to a full Senate investigation. And frankly, I think you ought to try your own medicine next time before you try to market it and put a positive spin on it.”

LaForge stiffened.

Gonzalez and Chen were in disbelief. They had caught the misdeed. But at what cost?

Thousands—maybe millions—of patients who had already taken Serovalta were unaware that they were losing pieces of themselves with each passing day. Some might recover, but others might never regain what had been stripped away. How many marriages had crumbled under the weight of emotional detachment? How many families had watched their once vibrant loved ones become hollow shells? And how much further had trust in medicine eroded?

Both doctors had spent her career believing in the ethical obligations of pharmaceutical companies and the adequacy of regulatory processes employed by the FDA, but tonight, as they walked out of the hearing room, neither was sure if they still did.

30. Dare to Touch

A doctor makes her case for hands-on training, knowing there are no shortcuts to good clinical practice.

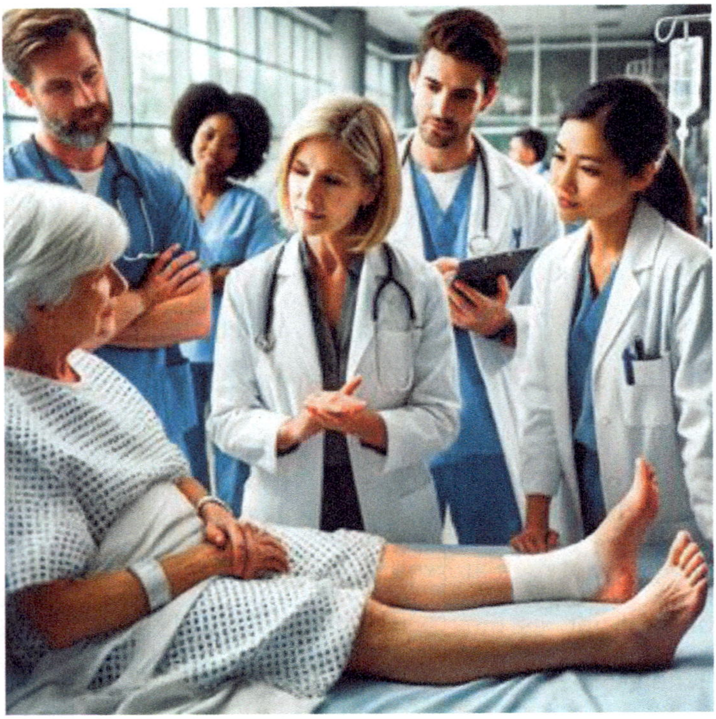

The AMC-affiliated community hospital brimmed with activity—nurses moving swiftly between patient rooms, residents huddled over charts, and the cadenced beeping of monitors echoing through the halls. Dr. Molly Wainwright led a group of third-year medical students through the ward on morning rounds, her steps purposeful, her tablet tucked under one arm. Ryan, one of the more eager students, walked beside her, though frustration was beginning to take root in his expression. Glenna, Ryan's always observant classmate, trailed slightly behind, absorbing the morning's lessons in silence.

Stopping outside a patient's room, Dr. Wainwright scanned her notes before pushing the door open. Inside, Mrs. Papadakis, a 72-year-old woman with uncontrolled diabetes, sat upright in bed, her foot propped on a pillow. Her skin was pale, but her eyes were sharp with curiosity as she regarded the white-coated group filing into her room.

"Good morning, Mrs. Papadakis," Dr. Wainwright bellowed, addressing her with a genuine smile. "I have several student doctors with me today. I hope that's alright." Not bothering to seek actual confirmation, Dr. Wainwright turned to Ryan. "Why don't you start by examining Mrs. Papadakis's foot and describing what you see?"

Ryan hesitated, shifting on his feet. "Uh, Dr. Wainwright… I was told we're only allowed to observe.

No hands-on patient care unless we're rotating at the AMC teaching—er, university—hospital."

She frowned, arms crossing over her chest. "Who made that policy and gave you the impression we were not a teaching hospital?"

"The hospital's HR department sent us a memo. Look, he said, producing it for her. It says students should strictly observe and never provide patient care."

Dr. Wainwright grabbed the memo, scanning it while Ryan continued.

"Even during our rotations at the university hospital, we're often just watching residents work. I haven't performed a real physical exam on a patient since I started clinicals."

Silence settled over the group. Some students nodded in agreement; others glanced at one another uneasily, unsure whether to confirm or deny Ryan's words. The burden of their shared frustration lingered in the room, an unspoken truth.

Dr. Wainwright was clearly annoyed. She took over and stepped closer to the bed. "Mrs. Papadakis, are you having any issues today?"

"Oh, you know, doctor," the woman said with a tired but warm smile, "just hoping this foot doesn't get any worse."

Dr. Wainwright's tone softened. "Would you be comfortable if Ryan examines your foot under my supervision?"

Mrs. Papadakis didn't bat an eyelash. "Of course not! How else will they learn? Go on, dear, take a look. I don't bite."

Ryan shot a glance at Dr. Wainwright, who gave him a slight nod. With a deep breath, he stepped forward, slipping on a pair of gloves before carefully lifting the woman's foot. He studied the ulcer on the plantar surface, noting the signs of infection—mild erythema, purulent drainage, and the faint telltale odor. His hands were steady, his mind engaged in a way it hadn't been in weeks.

"The ulcer is about two centimeters in diameter," he murmured, thinking aloud. "It looks like there's a possible infection."

Dr. Wainwright's voice was encouraging. "Good. What's your next step?"

He furrowed his brow. “I’d check for signs of osteomyelitis—maybe an X-ray or MRI?”

She nodded. “Exactly. And what about bedside tests?”

Ryan’s eyes brightened with realization. “The probe-to-bone test.”

A smile played at the edges of Dr. Wainwright’s lips. “That’s the kind of thinking we need. But you wouldn’t have made those connections if you had just observed, would you?”

Shaking his head, Ryan felt the weight of the moment settle over him. “No way. Reading about it isn’t the same as doing it. I feel like I actually know something now.”

Dr. Wainwright turned to the rest of the group, her voice carrying an unmistakable conviction. “Hospitals face pressures—risk management, efficiency, liability concerns—but if we continue down this path, we’ll have a generation of doctors who’ve never touched a patient before stepping into practice. Imagine walking into a hospital and being treated by a physician who has never placed a central line, never sutured a wound, never even palpated an abdomen. That’s not just bad education—it’s dangerous medicine.”

Glenna, quiet until now, furrowed her brows. “I get that institutions are worried about liability, but isn’t there a way to balance supervision with hands-on training? After all, our medical school has a connection to this hospital and others where we train.

Dr. Wainwright nodded. “That’s exactly the question we should be asking. We need engaged preceptors, structured supervision, and an acknowledgment that real training doesn’t happen behind a computer. Shadowing and simulation don’t make a doctor. Touching, feeling, listening—those do.”

A thoughtful silence settled over the group. Mrs. Papadakis reached out, patting Ryan’s hand with a gentle touch. “Doctors need to learn how to take care of people. Not just what they read in books, but people—real people who are patients—and not those dummies you practice on.”

Everyone had a good laugh. Dr. Wainwright smiled at her students, sensing the shift in their stance. They stood a little taller now, their expressions a little more resolute. They weren’t just observers anymore. They were learning—truly learning—to be doctors.

As they stepped into the hallway, the morning rounds continued, but something had changed. Medicine wasn't just an academic pursuit. It was a craft, an art—a human one. And it had to be protected.

***

That afternoon, Dr. Wainwright strode into the administrative wing of the hospital, her pulse steady but her determination unwavering. The sterile, fluorescent-lit corridor led to the HR office, where policy decisions were made in the interest of liability and efficiency—but rarely in the interest of education.

She knocked once before pushing the door open, catching the HR director, Ms. Collins, mid-email. The woman looked up, adjusting her glasses, and offered a tight smile. "Dr. Wainwright, what can I do for you?"

Without preamble, she placed a copy of the HR memo on the desk. "We need to talk about this."

Ms. Collins skimmed the document, her expression unreadable. "This policy is in place to minimize legal risks—"

"And it's undermining medical education," Dr. Wainwright interjected. "I just watched a third-year medical student examine a patient for the first time in months. Months, Ms. Collins. That is unacceptable."

Leaning forward, she continued, her voice even but firm. "We cannot train competent physicians if they are never given the opportunity to practice under supervision. If we continue down this path, we are sending graduates into residency with no real experience—setting them, and their future patients, up for failure. Worse yet, they will be rejected by residency programs for insufficient clinical experience."

Ms. Collins pursed her lips, considering. "The university has concerns about supervision ratios and liability—"

"That's why we have residents and attendings supervising. No one is asking for students to work unsupervised. But observation alone does not create doctors. It creates technicians who can recite facts but lack the ability to diagnose with their hands, to recognize subtleties, and to make clinical decisions in real time."

Ms. Collins sighed. "I admit, you're not the first to raise this concern."

"Then it's time we do something about it," Dr. Wainwright pressed. "I'm asking for a policy revision to allow students to conduct supervised exams and basic procedures, just as they did for decades before risk management began interfering with education."

There was a long pause before Ms. Collins nodded slowly. "I'll bring it up at the next administrative meeting."

"That's not enough," Dr. Wainwright said. "I want to advocate for such initiatives at all the AMC-affiliated hospitals where students rotate. If we don't act now, we'll regret it in a decade when we're working alongside physicians who were never truly trained."

Ms. Collins exhaled but finally nodded. "Alright. Let's start the discussion."

Dr. Wainwright stood, satisfied but far from finished. She had sparked a conversation—but now, she needed to turn it into action.

***

Several weeks later, Dr. Wainwright stood before a joint meeting of AMC executives, CEOs of affiliated community hospitals, and hospital administrators. At the head of the conference table sat the Dean of the medical school, who had taken a particular interest in the issue after hearing student complaints. The stakes were high, but Dr. Wainwright knew she wasn't alone in this fight.

Clearing her throat, she began. "We are failing our students. The hands-off policies enforced across our community hospitals have created a generation of future physicians who lack direct patient care experience. This is not just an educational issue—it's a patient safety issue. When students are denied hands-on experience, they enter residency without the fundamental skills necessary to provide safe and effective care. Without direct patient interaction, they fail to develop the ability to recognize subtle but critical clinical signs, delaying diagnoses and potentially leading to worse patient outcomes. Physicians who lack real-world training are more likely to make errors, misinterpret findings, and hesitate in high-stakes situations. This policy doesn't just hinder education—it places future patients at risk by sending out underprepared doctors into an already burdened healthcare system. You may think this policy ensures safety, but it actually worsens it."

The room was stone-cold silent for what seemed like an eternity, but gradually she began to see nods of agreement from some of the administrators. The Dean leaned forward, his hands clasped. “Dr. Wainwright is absolutely right. Our medical school cannot, in good conscience, continue to place students in rotations where they are observers rather than participants.”

One of the hospital CEOs adjusted his glasses. “Liability is a concern. If students make errors—”

The Dean cut him off. “Then they should make them under proper supervision, where they can learn. Residents were once students who had hands-on training. Did you know the ‘laying on of hands’ in medicine dates back centuries? Physical touch can lead to a diagnosis and promote healing. It conveys a deep sense of compassion and empathy. How do we expect students to be competent and compassionate if they never receive that experience?”

Dr. Wainwright pressed on. “I propose we reinstate supervised hands-on training across all AMC-affiliated hospitals. We must revise policies to allow students to conduct physical exams, perform basic procedures, and engage with patients under the direct supervision of residents and attendings.”

Silence followed, until another administrator finally spoke. The CEO of the mid-sized community hospital also cleared his throat and began to speak, his expression tense. "Let's not ignore the financial implications here. If we allow medical students to take on more hands-on responsibilities, our malpractice insurance rates will rise—not just for my hospital, but for all of them. Who is going to absorb that cost?"

The room shifted, a few murmurs rippling through the executives.

Dr. Wainwright met his gaze steadily. "I understand your concern, but let's consider the bigger picture. What's more costly—slightly higher insurance premiums now, or a generation of undertrained physicians making preventable mistakes later—possibly mistakes made in your hospital when that student decides to stay on for residency? If we invest in proper training now, we reduce long-term risks. Furthermore, many malpractice insurers recognize the value of structured supervision and education in reducing claims. If we implement a standardized training framework, we may be able to negotiate these concerns more effectively."

The Dean nodded in agreement. "And let's not forget the value of our partnerships. It's a win-win: the med students learn, and you have a ready-made pipeline of future doctors. No one wants to see these partnerships dissolve. We can explore funding options and shared liability strategies. Other teaching hospitals have managed to do this, and so can we. The alternative—sending unprepared doctors into practice—is far riskier in the long run."

The CEO sighed but gave a small nod. "Alright. But we need clear guidelines on supervision and documentation to keep liability manageable. This would require rewriting our agreements with the AMC."

The Dean nodded. "Then we rewrite them. Effective immediately, I am appointing a committee to draft new guidelines that will ensure our students are trained properly. And I will personally see to it that these changes are implemented across all affiliated sites."

A murmur spread through the room. Some administrators looked reluctant, but the tide was shifting. Finally, the CEO of the largest community hospital stood. "If this is the direction AMC is taking, we will support it. As for others in the room, I hope you join in. It's not only a win-win. I would say there is an intangible aspect to being a teaching hospital—prestige."

Dr. Wainwright exhaled, feeling the weight of victory settle over her. The battle wasn't over, but the momentum had shifted. Future doctors would no longer be sidelined. They would learn, hands-on, as they always should have.

As the meeting adjourned, the Dean turned to Dr. Wainwright with a smile. "Good work. You've just changed medical education for the better."

31. Second Act

Doctors may want to consider non-clinical career options—whether or not they're burned out.

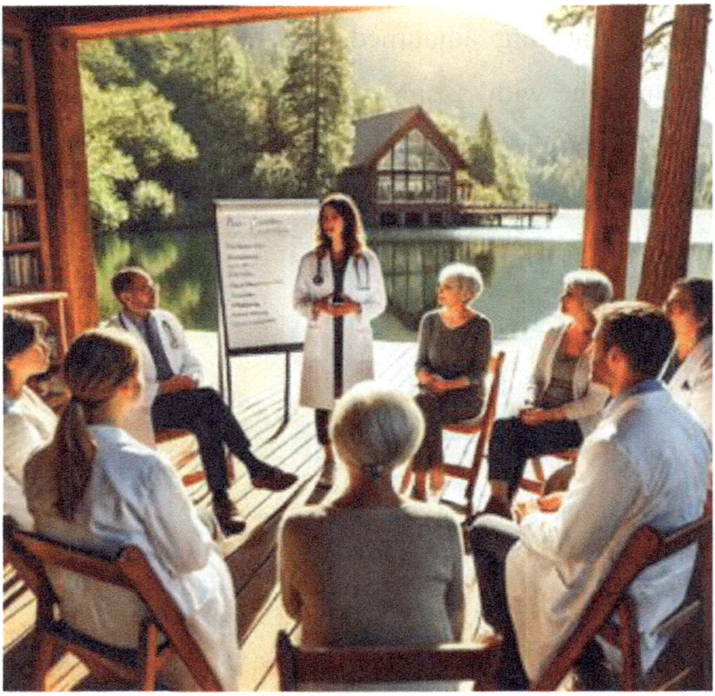

The message appeared late at night, just as Dr. Eliza Martin was about to close her laptop. She was a psychiatrist who had recovered from burnout—she liked to think of herself as a "recovering" physician—and now ran a coaching business for physicians in transition. Some were burned out like she was, some disillusioned, others simply lost. But this message wasn't about burnout. It was something darker, rawer.

"I've been in health care my entire life—Ob/Gyn. I spoke up about something I shouldn't have, and now I'm out of a job. Blacklisted. Fifty-seven years old, nothing to show for it. I buried everything—every ounce of pain—in my work. Now there's nothing but time, and I can't escape it. The thoughts...they don't stop. I think about ending it every single day. Some nights, the pull is unbearable. I cry myself to sleep more often than not. I don't want to live anymore."

Eliza sat up straighter. She had read thousands of messages over the years—doctors on the brink, physicians drowning in grief. But this one—it felt like a hand reaching from the edge of a cliff.

She typed quickly.

"I hear you. I see you. You are not alone. Please stay. Let's talk."

The reply came five minutes later.

"Disregard my note. I reread what I wrote—it just sounds like some pathetic pity party. But why does it feel so overwhelming? Why is the thought of ending things

always there? Why do I feel like I'd be better off dead? Some nights, I scratch my arms, just to feel something. The pain has taken everything. Even my faith. Even the strength I used to have."

Eliza exhaled, the weight of the words pressing into her chest. She had learned long ago, dealing with similar situations, not to panic, not to flinch.

She hesitated only a second before typing.

"You're not throwing a pity party. You're grieving. And you're not weak. You're carrying an impossible weight. Let me hold some of it with you."

For a long time, there was nothing. She stared at the screen, waiting, hoping. Then—an alert.

An unknown number. Anonymous.

She hesitated before answering. "Dr. Martin."

The voice on the other end was barely above a whisper. "I don't know why I called."

"Yes, you do," Eliza said gently. "Because you want to be heard."

A shaky breath. Then, "I feel disposable. Like I never existed."

She let the silence stretch. "You're here. Talking to me. That means something."

A bitter laugh. "It means I've run out of options."

"No. It means you're still fighting."

"I don't feel like I am."

"You are. Calling me? That's fighting. Putting words to the pain? That's fighting."

A pause. "It doesn't change anything, though."

Eliza leaned back in her chair, closing her eyes. "Maybe not tonight. But let's talk anyway."

A sigh on the other end. "I lost everything. I fought for my patients—abortion rights—and it cost me my career. And the worst part? I have no one. My kids are grown. I'm divorced. My parents are gone. I just…worked. And now, without the work, there's nothing left."

Eliza swallowed. She had seen it before. Physicians who built their lives around service until, one day, the scaffolding collapsed. "You spent years caring for others and saving lives. But no one ever taught you how to save your own."

A sharp inhale. "How the hell am I supposed to do that now?"

"One breath at a time," Eliza said. "One conversation at a time. One act of care—for yourself—at a time."

Silence.

Then—"I don't know how."

"That's okay. I'll help you figure it out."

A long pause. Then, quieter, "I still don't know if it matters."

"It does."

Another silence. Then—softer—"I don't think I can promise I won't think about it. The darkness is always there."

"I understand," Eliza said. "But can you promise me this? Stay tonight. Call me tomorrow. Just one more day."

A breath. A long exhale.

"…Yeah. Okay."

"Good," she said, voice steady. "Then that's enough for now."

Eliza let out a breath she hadn't realized she was holding—a breath of relief. She was willing to bet her phone would ring tomorrow. She didn't like being cast into the role of a lifeline once more, a role she had thought she left behind. Yet, beneath the discomfort of being thrust back into clinical action, she felt a familiar sense of purpose. The urgency of the caller's situation reignited a spark within her—a reminder of why she had chosen this path in the first place. As she hung up the phone, Eliza resolved to stay by the caller's side, if only metaphorically, and to use every skill she had honed over the years to guide her through the darkness. Tomorrow, she thought, would be a new opportunity to help someone find their way back to hope.

***

Eliza's phone buzzed just past noon the next day. She had been expecting it.

She answered on the first ring. "Dr. Martin."

A pause. Then, "It's me." The voice was steadier this time.

Eliza smiled to herself. "I'm glad you called."

A heavy sigh. "I almost didn't. Woke up feeling like…what's the point?"

"But you called anyway," Eliza noted. "That's the point."

There was silence between them until the caller finally spoke again. "I need to get out of this hole."

"You will," Eliza said firmly. "But not alone. Have you thought about seeing someone? A therapist?"

A shaky breath. "Yeah. I looked up a few names last night. Made an appointment."

Relief flooded Eliza's chest. She knew that being able to think about the future was a good sign. "Good. That's the next step."

"I don't know if it'll help."

"It will. If you let it."

Another pause. "I don't know what comes next for me."

"We don't need to figure that out today," Eliza said gently. "Right now, the focus is on keeping you safe and getting support. We'll tackle the rest later."

"Okay." The word was soft, but it carried a weight of acceptance—not defeat.

Eliza leaned forward in her chair. “I need to ask you something.”

A long pause. “I know what you’re going to ask.”

“Are you still thinking about ending it?”

Another pause. Then — “No.”

Eliza closed her eyes briefly, exhaling. “I need you to promise me something.”

“What?”

“That if that feeling creeps back in, you’ll reach out. To your therapist, to me, to a friend, to a crisis resource. You won’t sit with it alone.”

“Yeah,” the voice was hoarse. “I promise.”

“Good,” Eliza said. “I want to make sure you have some resources on hand as well. Can you grab a pen?”

There was a rustling sound. “Got one.”

Eliza began listing. “First—988. That’s the suicide and crisis lifeline. It’s there 24/7.”

“Got it.”

"Your local medical society—many have physician support programs. It's worth checking out, but make sure you stay 'anonymous'—no pun intended."

A giggle. Another good sign. "But…why anonymous?"

"Because unfortunately participating in physician health programs can cause obstacles if you decide to re-enter practice. So, make sure if you choose to go that route, you can be guaranteed confidentiality."

"Now…The Lorna Breen Heroes' Foundation. They help physicians dealing with burnout and mental health crises."

A slow breath. "Didn't even know that existed."

"Most don't," Eliza said. "But it's there. It was founded to honor a true hero, a doctor who succumbed to the emotional toll of COVID when the system failed her. Google the website and check it out."

She hesitated, then added, "And there's always me. My number, my email. If things get bad, reach out again."

Silence. Then—"You don't even know me."

"I don't have to," Eliza said. "You're a doctor. You've given your life to taking care of others. Now it's your turn to be taken care of."

Another pause. Then, quietly, "Thank you."

Eliza smiled. “One more thing.”

“What?”

“I run a retreat for doctors figuring out their next steps. It’s not therapy, but it’s a place to breathe. To be among like-minded physicians who are also trying to figure things out. To think about what’s next—when you’re ready.”

A dry chuckle. “Not sure I’m retreat material.”

“No one thinks they are,” Eliza said. “But when you are ready…consider it.”

A breath. Then, “I will.”

Eliza let the silence settle before saying, “You did something important today.”

“What’s that?”

“You stayed.”

A pause. Then, softly, “Yeah. I did.”

And for the first time, Eliza believed the voice on the other end of the line was starting to believe it, too.

***

The sun hung low over the retreat center, casting long shadows across the deck where a handful of physicians sat nursing their coffee and soda and quietly murmuring among themselves. Dr. Eliza Martin watched the group from a distance, recognizing the weary postures and the half-hopeful, half-skeptical expressions. She had seen this before—physicians arriving at her retreats carrying the weight of loss, uncertainty, and burnout. Some came to heal. Some came searching for escape.

And some—some just wanted to see if anything could make them feel human again.

"Eliza."

The voice was low but steady. She turned.

A woman stood a few feet away, shifting a canvas bag over one shoulder. Her hair was turning grey, her frame lean in the way that suggested decades of long hours on her feet. The eyes, though—Eliza had imagined those eyes before the name even came.

"I'm Dr. Marjorie Taylor." A pause. "I was the caller..."

Eliza felt her breath hitch.

Marjorie smiled—small but real. "I thought it was time to introduce myself properly."

Eliza's chest tightened, but she smiled back. "I'm so glad you're here."

They stepped away from the others, settling into two Adirondack chairs overlooking the lake.

"How are you?" Eliza asked, studying her carefully.

Marjorie exhaled. "Better," she said. "I'm in therapy. I also see a psychiatrist for antidepressants. No shame in that—right? And before you ask—no, I don't think about dying every day anymore." She looked out at the water. "I still have rough days, but I don't feel alone in them. That makes all the difference."

Eliza felt something unclench in her chest. "I can't tell you how relieved I am to hear that."

Marjorie chuckled. "Yeah, me too." She tapped her fingers against her knee. "So, I'm here because I want to figure out what the heck I'm going to do with the rest of my life. The clinical doors are closed. I'm trying to see what's on the other side."

Eliza nodded. "You came to the right place."

A bell rang in the distance, signaling the next session. The two of them made their way inside, joining the other physicians who had gathered in a circle of chairs.

Eliza stood at the front. “So, let’s talk about why you’re here,” she said. “For most of us, medicine was the plan. And now, for whatever reason, it’s not. Maybe you were forced out. Maybe you walked away. Maybe you’re just figuring out if you need an exit plan. But the reality is—there is life beyond clinical practice. And I want us to talk about what that can look like.”

She glanced around the room. “Let’s start with this. How many of you have seriously considered a non-clinical career before?”

A few hands went up hesitantly.

A man in the back spoke spontaneously. “I guess I have, but it always felt…like giving up. Like, if I wasn’t practicing, then what was I even doing with my degree?”

Marjorie spoke next, before she could stop herself. “You’re existing,” she said. “Which is more than some of us thought we’d be doing a few months ago.”

The room went still for a while. Eliza watched as heads turned toward Marjorie with quiet curiosity.

She shrugged. "Sorry. Didn't mean to lay that on you and hijack the conversation. It's just… I spent my whole life thinking my OB career was my identity. Then I lost it, and I thought I lost me. But I didn't. I just had no idea who I was outside of the delivery room."

A woman across from her leaned forward. "So, how do you start over? What are the actual options?"

Eliza gestured toward a whiteboard. "Let's start with the big-ticket items and break it down." She started writing:

Non-Clinical Career Options for Physicians

I. **Medical Writing & Journalism**— "For those of you who love explaining complex topics to people, medical writing can be a great path. You can write for medical journals, consumer health sites, or even do copywriting for biotech companies."

II. **Consulting & Pharma**—"Industry work is huge. Pharma, biotech, and device companies—they all need doctors for clinical strategy, regulatory affairs, and safety and medical science liaison roles."

III. **Coaching & Leadership Development**—"Some of you, like me, may want to coach other physicians. Leadership development, burnout coaching, and executive coaching—these are all growing fields."

IV. **Health Tech & AI** —"For the tech-savvy among you, there are tons of roles in digital health, AI applications in medicine, and product development."

V. **Legal & Expert Witness Work** —"Some "doctors go into medical-legal consulting, working on cases of malpractice, disability evaluations, or forensic medicine."

VI. **Teaching & Academia** —"Not every doctor wants to leave medicine entirely. Teaching, curriculum development, or mentoring medical students can be a fulfilling path."

VII. **Public Health & Policy** —"For those of you interested in making systemic change, public health leadership, working with the WHO, CDC, or nonprofits, can be incredibly impactful."

She turned back to the group. "So, what jumps out at you?"

The man from earlier rubbed his chin. "I never thought about pharma. I mean, I hate the politics of it, but it's probably the most stable of these. And I heard you don't need previous industry experience for some jobs."

The woman who had asked about starting over nodded toward 'Coaching & Leadership.' "I don't know, I've spent so many years mentoring residents. Maybe there's something in that?"

Eliza smiled. "Exactly. The trick isn't just finding a job. It's finding a job that mirrors what you loved about clinical work—without the parts that broke you."

She glanced at Marjorie, who was quiet, scanning the list.

Eliza nudged her. "Anything stand out?"

Marjorie hesitated. "The writing part."

Eliza raised a brow.

Marjorie shrugged. "I used to write. Years ago. But it wasn't…medical. It was more personal stuff."

Eliza grinned. "So? The world needs more personal stuff from doctors who've lived it."

Marjorie exhaled, a small, wry smile forming. "Guess I have a few stories to tell."

Eliza nodded. "Then tell them."

The room was quiet again, but this time, it wasn't heavy. It was the quiet of gears turning, possibilities forming.

For the first time in a long time, Marjorie Taylor didn't feel anonymous.

She felt like a woman with a future.

32. This Note's for You

A psychiatry resident learns that mistakes are inevitable. It's what comes next that counts.

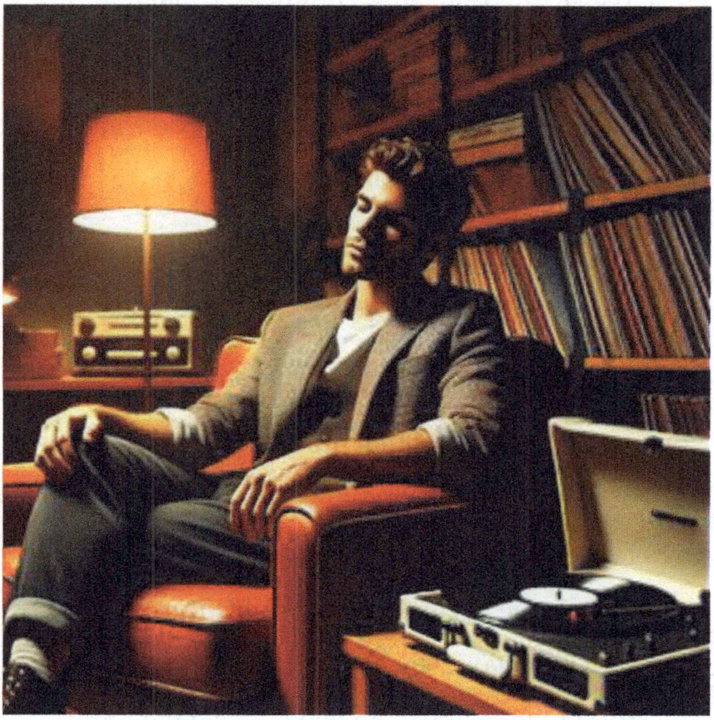

Psychiatry resident Zach Miller stared at his reflection in the glass of his office window, his stomach still tight from the morning's session. The words replayed in his head like a song stuck on repeat, an off-key note he couldn't unhear.

"You just don't get it, do you?"

His patient, Kevin, had been in the middle of a vulnerable moment—talking about the crushing weight of loneliness after his divorce. And what had Zach done? He'd reached for a silver lining too soon, trying to lighten the pain instead of sitting with it.

"You've still got time to rebuild—" he had said, before Kevin cut him off with that hard stare.

Zach had seen the flicker of disappointment— the subtle withdrawal. He had stepped on something fragile, something Kevin hadn't been ready to let go of.

Now, hours later, he still felt the embarrassment coursing through him, a heat behind his ears. He had studied for years for this—read every major book, analyzed relevant case studies, and spent sleepless nights preparing for the gravity of this work, this work we call psychotherapy. And still, in the moment, he had misread the room.

"If I'm making mistakes like this now, what happens when it matters more, when someone's life is literally at stake?"

The thought was suffocating. He took a deep breath, trying to steady the rising tide of self-doubt. It was a reminder, albeit a harsh one, of the immense responsibility he bore. Yet, he knew that growth often came from these uncomfortable moments. With each misstep, there was an opportunity to learn, to recalibrate, and to become a better clinician. He resolved to seek guidance from his supervisor to dissect where he had gone wrong and how he could improve.

Just then, fortuitously, a knock at the door jolted him.

Dr. Tobias Troyer stepped in without waiting for a reply, a well-worn leather satchel slung over his shoulder, the odd smell of aged cheese and apple slices clinging to his trademark turtleneck sweater. Toby—everyone called him that—was a legend in the department. Patients adored him, residents hung onto his every word, and he had a way of making even the most lost causes seem salvageable, as well as the residents who butchered them.

He also had an uncanny way of reading people.

"You're brooding." Toby tossed his satchel onto the chair opposite Zach's desk and perched on the edge of it. "Let me guess. A session went sideways?"

Zach hesitated before nodding. “More south than sideways. Kevin. I said the wrong thing. Pushed the hope button too soon. He shut down.”

Toby nodded, as if he could already hear the whole conversation in his head. “And now you’re spiraling, wondering if this means you’re a fraud, doomed to make a string of catastrophic mistakes until someone realizes you’re not fit to practice?”

Zach threw his hands up. “Well, I wasn’t thinking of all that—until now.”

Toby grinned and leaned back. “Let me tell you something. You know who else made mistakes like that?”

Zach tilted his head. “Who?”

“Me.” Toby stretched his legs out, crossing his ankles. “I once had a patient tell me I was the most unhelpful psychiatrist he’d ever had. And guess what?”

“What?”

“He wasn’t wrong.”

Zach’s eyes sparkled.

Toby chuckled. “Early in my career, I thought my job was to fix things. Give solutions. Offer perspective. Turns out, people don’t always want that. Sometimes, they just want someone to sit in the wreckage with them.”

“That’s exactly it.” Zach sat forward. “I know that. I just…forgot. And now I feel like I broke something in the relationship.”

Toby shook his head. “You know Miles Davis once said, ‘It’s not the note you play that’s the wrong note—it’s the note you play afterwards that makes it right or wrong.’”

Zach frowned. “Are you saying my rookie mistake is just jazz improvisation?”

Toby grinned. “Something like that.” He tapped his fingers on Zach’s desk, drumming an imaginary rhythm. “Therapy’s the same way. We will hit wrong notes. That’s inevitable. What matters is what comes next.”

Zach leaned back, letting the words settle.

“You’re going to repair this,” Toby continued. “You’ll acknowledge what happened. You’ll sit with it. And Kevin? He’ll appreciate that more than if you had gotten everything right the first time.”

Zach exhaled, some of the tension loosening in his chest. “So, you’re saying I didn’t ruin the whole symphony?”

Toby chuckled. “Nah. You just played a note that needed some resolving.”

Zach smirked. “You really believe in this whole music metaphor, huh?”

Toby shrugged. “What can I say? It works.” He stood, grabbing his satchel. “Now go make it right. And in the meantime, maybe put on some good jazz tonight and remind yourself—mistakes aren’t the end of the song. They’re just part of the music.”

As Toby left, Zach turned back to his reflection in the window.

The mistake still stung, but maybe—just by chance—it wasn’t the wrong note after all.

Maybe it was just the setup for something better.

***

Later that night, Zach sank into the old leather chair in his apartment, the one that had somehow followed him from med school to residency, its worn arms proof of every late-night study session and crisis of confidence he had ever had.

His dad's vinyl collection sat neatly stacked beside him, a relic from a different era—one where music wasn't just background noise but something you listened to—like listening to patients— something that filled the room and pressed itself into your bones, just like the needle had pressed itself into the vinyl grooves, creating those unmistakable "snap, crackle, and pops" now sanitized by digital reissues.

Tonight, he needed the original.

He thumbed through the albums, skipping past the classics his dad would have reached for—Springsteen, Van Morrison, Steely Dan, the Grateful Dead—the ones he'd researched on eBay and Discogs to see how much money they fetched. His fingers finally landed on a familiar sleeve. Neil Young—This Note's for You.

He smiled. His dad had loved Neil Young—still does—always talking about how the guy refused to sell out, refused to let anyone dictate his sound. Authenticity, that was the word his dad used. Neil played what was true to him, whether people liked it or not. Young was the real reason his dad schlepped Zach to see CSN&Y perform during their 2006 “Freedom of Speech” reunion tour. Young’s bandmates were okay, but Young…was the fire—the unrelenting force that made the performance feel urgent, raw, and necessary. His voice, weathered but fierce, carried the weight of conviction, and his guitar work cut through the air like a call to arms. While the rest of CSN&Y delivered nostalgia, Young delivered a reckoning.

Zach slid the record from its sleeve, set the needle, and let the first notes wail through the speakers.

“Don’t want no cash, don’t need no money

Ain’t got no stash; this note’s for you...”

The brass section came in, warm and brash, a sound that refused to be ignored.

Zach let the music wash over him, absorbing its defiant energy. This note’s for you.

For the first time all day, he let go of the loop playing in his head—the worry, the doubt, the endless picking apart of his mistake. He realized now that therapy, much like music, wasn’t about playing every note perfectly. It was about feeling it, about staying true to the moment, about trusting that even the missteps had their place in the rhythm.

He thought about what Toby had said.

“It’s not the note you play that’s the wrong note—it’s the note you play afterwards that makes it right or wrong.”

Zach smiled to himself, resting his head back against the chair.

He could still hear Kevin’s voice, the disappointment in it. But now, instead of dreading their next session, he found himself looking forward to it.

Not to fix what had happened.

But to own it. And move on.

To keep playing.

The record spun, the horn section blaring unapologetically, as Zach let himself settle into something new — something that felt a hell of a lot like freedom: to create his artistic oeuvre as a psychotherapist.

33. The Tremor

A physician becomes a patient.

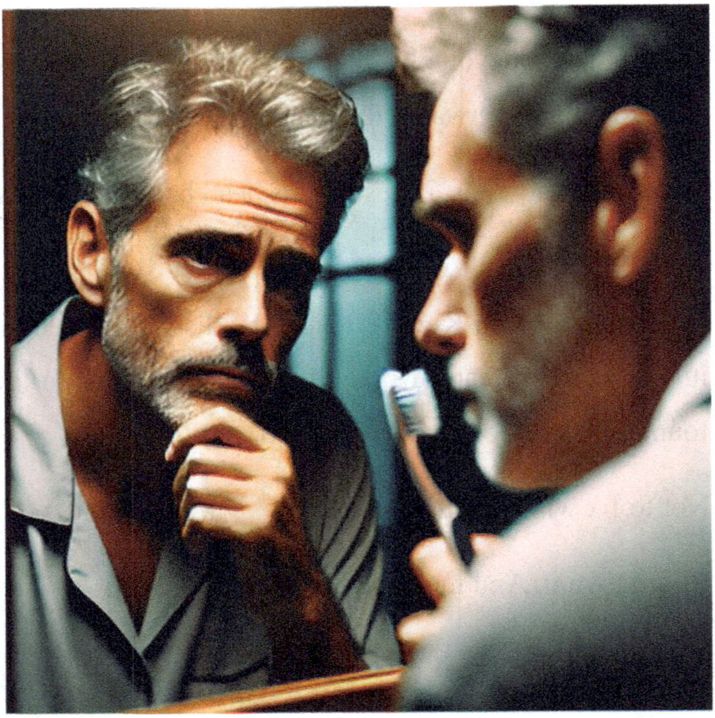

Dr. Daniel Mercer had spent three decades studying the brain's intricate mysteries, peering at neuronal pathways under the glow of fluorescence microscopes, and pushing the frontiers of research into neurodegenerative diseases. He had written groundbreaking papers on Parkinson's disease, lectured at the world's finest institutions, and sat on advisory boards for clinical trials.

Needless to say, his expertise as a neurologist—a specialist in movement disorders—was highly regarded and sought after.

Yet now, standing in front of a mirror, he couldn't deny what he had been trying to ignore for months.

His right hand trembled ever so slightly as he reached for his toothbrush.

It wasn't fatigue. It wasn't stress. It wasn't a fluke.

He clenched and unclenched his fist, as if he could will it away. The movement was barely perceptible, but he knew better than anyone what it meant.

Denial became his first line of defense. He worked harder, longer, and avoided extended conversations with colleagues who might notice the subtle hesitations in his movements. He convinced himself it was nothing.

Then came the stiffness in his right leg. The slowness of his steps. The slight hesitation before turning a corner.

One evening, at a department gala, his wife, Helen, reached for his hand beneath the linen-draped table.

"Danny," she whispered, squeezing gently, "your hand is shaking."

He pulled away instinctively. He forced a smile. “Maybe I’m just excited about giving the keynote speech.”

Helen held his gaze longer than he wanted. “I know what it looks like,” she said softly, giving Daniel an opening to acknowledge what they both feared.

But he deflected as he felt his throat tighten. “Just too much coffee.”

The second line of defense was secrecy.

For months, he continued his research at the institute, hiding his growing difficulties. He made excuses when colleagues asked why he was walking more slowly or why his handwriting—once meticulous—now looked erratic on the whiteboard.

Then one morning, during “Professor’s” rounds at the hospital, he attempted to demonstrate a clinical exam on a patient with advanced Parkinson’s.

“Now, you’ll notice,” he said, slowly flexing and extending the patient’s arm at the elbow, “the classic cogwheel rigidity—"

His own hand trembled visibly.

The room fell silent. His residents, fellows, and peers stared at him. Dr. Eugene ("Gene") Smedley, his longtime colleague, shifted uncomfortably.

"Daniel," Gene murmured after the session, pulling him aside, "I think we need to talk."

Daniel straightened, feigning ignorance. "Talk about what?"

"You know what."

His hands were in his pockets, but the tremor persisted. Gene waited, giving him space, letting him come to it on his own.

Finally, Daniel exhaled, his shoulders slumping. "I didn't want to believe it."

"You have to let someone help you," Gene said. "You know as well as anyone, early intervention makes a difference."

"Help me?" Daniel scoffed bitterly. "I am the expert on Parkinson's. I've treated patients for years. I've dedicated my life to fighting this disease." He turned away. "And now I am the disease."

Gene placed a hand on his shoulder. “Danny, you’ve always been brilliant. But right now, you’re an idiot. None of us are immune to the diseases we study. There’s no shame in it.”

Daniel gave a short, humorless laugh. “I suppose I deserved being called an idiot.”

“Let me treat you.”

The words struck like a hammer. For years, Daniel had been the one diagnosing, advising, and comforting. The idea of surrendering his own care to someone else—it felt like an admission of failure.

But he knew the alternative.

***

A week later, he sat in Gene’s office as a patient.

Gene examined him with the same methodical precision Daniel himself had once used.

“You’re still in the early stages,” Gene said, sitting down across from him. “We have options.”

Daniel let out a slow breath. “You think I’ll make a good patient?”

Gene smirked. "You're already a pain in the ass."

They both chuckled, the tension breaking for the first time in months.

As treatment began, Daniel adapted. The tremor was there, but medication helped. He became more mindful of his movements, modifying his routine. His research continued—though at a different pace. He no longer saw himself as invincible—or as an embarrassment—but neither was he a victim.

Then came the surprise.

One evening, Helen handed him a thick envelope. "It came in today."

Daniel pursed his lips, opening them.

Inside was a research grant proposal, approved by the NIH. One of his own graduate students had submitted it under his mentorship.

His eyes scanned the project title:

"The Mercer Initiative: A Novel Approach to Parkinson's Disease Treatment."

He tried to catch his breath. The research he had once led was continuing—without him at the helm, but because of him.

And then, he read the specifics.

It was something he had theorized about years ago but dismissed as too ambitious: an experimental therapy using personalized, gene-edited stem cells derived from a patient's own skin cells, designed to replace damaged dopamine-producing neurons. Unlike conventional stem cell therapies, these cells would be pre-engineered to survive in the hostile neurodegenerative environment of a Parkinsonian brain.

It wasn't just another clinical trial. It was the trial.

Gene's name was on the proposal as a co-investigator.

Daniel swallowed hard. He knew what this meant.

One day—perhaps sooner than he wished—he would be a patient in that trial.

For a long time, he had feared that Parkinson's would rob him of everything.

But now, reading the proposal under the soft glow of his desk lamp, he realized something.

He wouldn't live to see the end of Parkinson's. But maybe it was possible he had helped push the first domino that would lead to its fall.

And for the first time since his diagnosis, he felt something unfamiliar.

Hope.

And pride.

34. A Eulogy for Medicine

A doctor contemplates narrative medicine writing as a remedy for a profession in mourning.

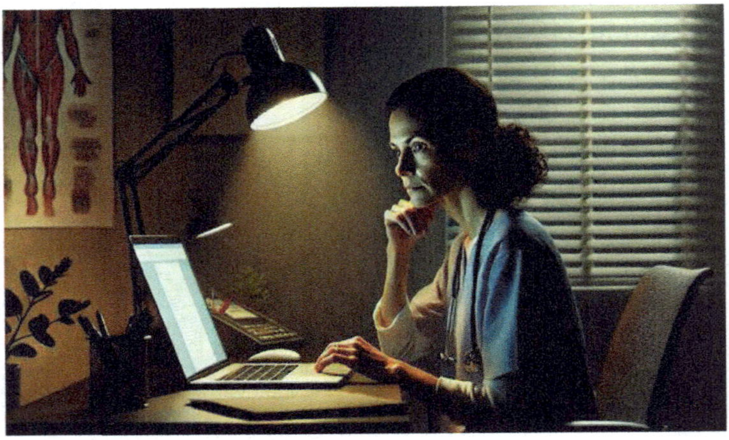

Dr. Grace Theobald sat at her desk, fingers hovering over the keyboard, staring at the blinking cursor that mocked her hesitation. The assignment from Professor Deborah ("Deb") Price-Gardner, her instructor for "Introduction to Narrative Medicine," was straightforward—write a eulogy for medicine. But how does one eulogize something that still breathes, still moves, yet feels irreparably wounded?

She exhaled sharply and began to type.

We are gathered here today to mourn the passing of medicine—not in the biological sense, but in spirit, in essence. Medicine, once a noble calling, a sacred duty, has withered under the weight of its own contradictions. We remember its early days, when the healer was a figure of reverence, when the act of tending to the sick was a covenant between knowledge and compassion. In those days, a physician's hands held the power to mend bodies, and their words held the power to brighten spirits.

But time has not been kind. The healer became the provider. The patient became the consumer. Those in need of counseling became clients. And medicine, once the devoted servant of human suffering, was placed on the auction block, bartered away in a labyrinth of administrators and insurers who had never smelled the metallic tang of fresh blood in an emergency room or witnessed the gray pallor of a failing heart. Medicine's decline was slow and insidious. It died not with a single blow, but with a thousand paper cuts—denials of necessary treatment, algorithms that overruled human judgment, quotas that rewarded speed over thoroughness, and profit margins that eclipsed patient outcomes.

For those who loved it, Medicine's death came with grief too complex for words. It was the grief of the young intern, watching their idealism erode under the relentless march of bureaucracy. It was the grief of the seasoned doctor, once alight with purpose, now exhausted and disillusioned. It was the grief of knowing that the work still needed to be done, but that the spirit in which it was once done had been lost.

And so, we stand here, witnesses to an era that is no more. The loss is incalculable. Medicine is survived by its estranged relatives—Technology, Efficiency, and Litigation—all of whom hold power in its absence but none of whom understand its soul. It leaves behind millions who still seek its wisdom, who still whisper their prayers to it in waiting rooms, hoping for something more than transactional healing. We, who once took an oath to do no harm, now find ourselves wondering: Was it medicine that was harmed beyond repair? Or was it we who did the harming by failing to recognize its demise—and intervene?

Rest in peace, Medicine. You deserved better.

Grace finished typing and leaned back in her chair. She closed her eyes. The words felt raw, almost too personal.

Maybe they were. Maybe they exposed something she wasn't quite ready to admit—that she, too, was grieving. That the frustration, the exhaustion, and the deep, aching disillusionment she had pushed aside for years had finally crystallized into something she could no longer ignore. She had written about the death of medicine, but in doing so, she had uncovered something else entirely—her own slow, creeping departure from it. The thought left a hollow ache in her chest. She opened her eyes and stared at the screen, uncertain whether she had written a eulogy for a profession or for a part of herself.

***

The following week, Grace arrived early at the local university and took her usual seat in the classroom. She silently deliberated whether to pursue other writing courses or simply be done with it once this course was over. If writing piqued her interest, she could obtain a "certificate" after three additional courses, or she could dive into a full-scale MFA program. She would wait to see how this one turned out.

Her printed eulogy rested on her desk like a fragile artifact. The room held a mix of professionals—

journalists, teachers, a few fellow physicians, and a retired lawyer who fancied himself the next Hemingway.

Deb smiled as she glanced around. “Grace, would you mind reading your piece?”

Grace hesitated, then nodded. She sat nervously and began. As she read, the room grew still, the usual scribbling of notes and shifting in chairs replaced by a quiet tension. When she finished, she folded the paper and looked up, bracing herself.

For a moment, silence. Then—

“Damn,” muttered a man in the back, a cardiologist named Peter. “That was brutal.”

Deb chuckled. “Brutal in a good way or a bad way?”

“Good. But depressing as hell.”

“I don’t think it’s depressing,” countered Shoshana, a former ER nurse turned budding novelist. “It’s just…honest.”

“It’s bleak,” said Shiv, a journalist. “But I get it. It reminds me of how war correspondents talk about journalism—how they start with this sense of duty, but after years in the trenches, they can't tell if they're making a difference anymore."

"You know what it reminds me of?" said Nora, a general surgeon. "Burnout surveys." She turned to Grace. "Did you write this from personal experience?"

Grace hesitated. "Not entirely. But I've felt pieces of it. I think most of us in medicine have."

A man who hadn't spoken yet, Thomas, a psychiatrist, rubbed his chin thoughtfully. "It reads more like bereavement than grief," explaining that grief is an emotional response to loss, while bereavement is the process of learning to live in the absence of what was lost. "Your piece doesn't just mourn medicine—it acknowledges that we are now forced to continue in its absence, adjusting to a reality where the ideals we once held no longer exist in the same way."

Deb jumped in. "Great insight. Grace, do you see this piece as a farewell or as a way of processing something ongoing?"

Grace sighed. "I think it's both. A farewell to what I thought medicine was, but also an attempt to make sense of what's left."

Peter nodded. “That’s exactly it. Medicine isn’t dead, but it’s…something else now. Something we have to figure out how to navigate.”

Deb smiled. “Let’s do this. For next week’s assignment, I want each of you to write a response to Grace’s eulogy. You can agree, disagree, challenge it, expand on it—whatever feels true to you. What do you see as the future of medicine? Hopeful, cynical, or somewhere in between?”

She smiled at Grace. “And Grace, excellent work. This was powerful. Hard to hear, but important.”

Grace nodded, still absorbing the room’s reaction. She had expected criticism. She hadn’t expected a conversation this layered and engaged. Maybe this class wasn’t just about writing.

Maybe it was about rediscovering what medicine could still be.

And if it required additional courses to find the answer, Grace was all in.

35. Out-of-Network, Out-of-Options, Out-of-Sorts

A patient needs urgent health care—and a doctor who will go to bat for her.

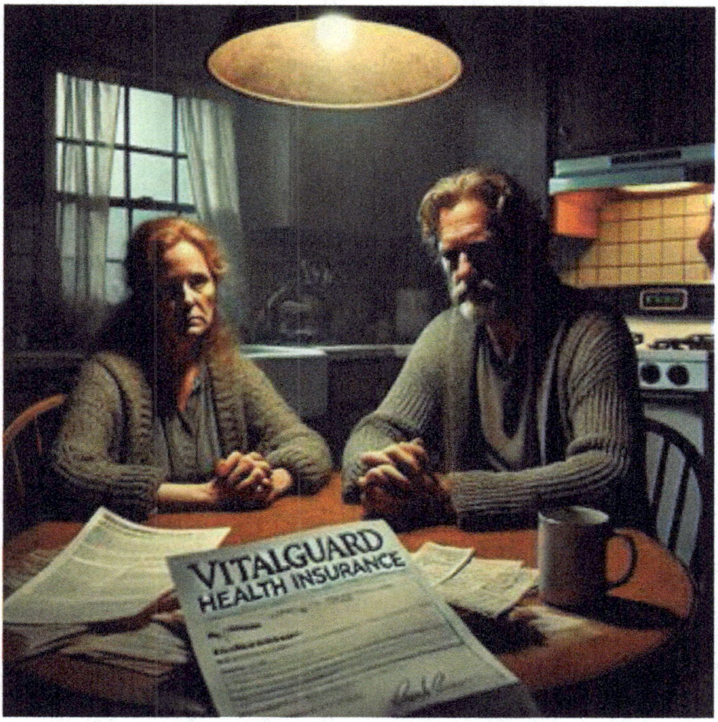

Sadie Cross sat at the kitchen table, staring at the letter in her trembling hands. The official blue-and-white letterhead of VitalGuard Health Insurance glared back at her, sterile and indifferent. The words blurred, but she had already memorized them.

"We understand that this news may cause you concern, and we want to reassure our customers that we remain committed to providing high-quality care."

Committed. Right. Customer. Not a patient.

Herb Cross leaned against the counter, arms folded, watching her. "What the hell does that even mean?" he asked, his voice tight with frustration.

Sadie swallowed hard. "It means that, after six months of covered treatment at Wilkerson Medical Center, they've suddenly decided that my surgery is out-of-network. They won't pay for it."

Herb rubbed a hand over his face. "That's insane. You've been seeing their specialists this whole time. They covered every MRI, every biopsy, and every pre-op test. And now, when it actually matters—"

"They pull the plug," Sadie finished. "Like it's just business as usual—not vital to them and not guarding over me."

Herb slammed his palm on the table. "Because it is business to them! We're just numbers, Sadie. They don't care if you live or die."

Sadie exhaled shakily. “Well, I care. Dr. Liao is the only surgeon in this area who’s done this procedure successfully more than a handful of times. If I wait months for VitalGuard and Wilkerson to work out a contract, I might not make it. And no other hospital even offers this surgery.”

Herb’s eyes darted to the stack of unpaid bills beside her. “How much would it cost out-of-pocket?”

Sadie closed her eyes. “Three hundred and forty thousand dollars.”

Silence.

Finally, Herb muttered, “That’s more than our house is worth.”

Sadie laughed bitterly. “Well, at least we wouldn’t have to worry about where I’d recover.”

Herb knelt beside her chair, gripping her hands. “I’ll sell the damn house, Sadie. I’ll do whatever it takes.”

She shook her head. “Even if we could pull together the money, I can’t stomach giving it to these leeches. I already paid for insurance. They should be covering this.”

Herb exhaled sharply. "Then we fight."

Sadie dropped the letter onto the pile of insurance statements. "How? Appeal? Already denied. Public pressure? VitalGuard will just say the same corporate garbage they always do. We don't have time to sue. And meanwhile, some CEO in a penthouse just signed off on my death sentence."

A heavy silence filled the room. Then Herb whispered, "What about Liao?"

Sadie was unsure. "What about him?"

Herb sat back on his heels. "He's top-tier. Big name. Hospitals compete for people like him. Maybe he has some kind of pull."

Sadie barked. "He's a surgeon, not a miracle worker."

Herb's jaw tightened. "Maybe. But we're out of options. So, let's see if he's willing to make some noise."

***

Dr. James Liao read Sadie's message three times before setting his phone down.

He wasn't surprised. This was happening more and more. Wilkerson Medical Center's contract negotiations with VitalGuard Health had stalled, leaving thousands of patients in limbo. But Sadie's case—it struck a nerve. He had spent months overseeing her care. He knew her, not just as a diagnosis but as a person. And now, thanks to bureaucratic nonsense, she might not get the surgery that could save her life.

Liao drummed his fingers against his desk, deep in thought. There was one card he hadn't played yet, one he had never intended to pony up.

Grabbing his phone, he dialed Charles Stillson, the hospital's CEO. The call was answered within seconds.

"James," Stillson greeted, his voice full of forced warmth. "I hope you're not calling about another budget request."

"I'm calling about Sadie Cross."

A beat. "Ah. Yes. Unfortunate situation. I heard."

"Unfortunate?" Liao yelled. "That's an interesting way to describe telling a patient they're out of luck because you and some VitalGuard executives can't agree on a reimbursement rate."

"James," Stillson said smoothly, "these negotiations take time. We're working in good faith."

"She doesn't have time."

Stillson paused. "We could consider a one-time exception for Ms. Cross."

Liao's stomach muscles tightened. "A special exception? So, you're fine letting every other patient in her position suffer, but because I raised hell, she gets a golden ticket?"

The silence was telling.

"No," Liao said flatly. "Not good enough."

"What are you proposing?"

"I'm proposing you finalize a contract with VitalGuard. Immediately."

Stillson let out a short laugh. "You think it's that simple? These deals take months."

Liao leaned back in his chair. "Maybe. But if you don't, I'll perform Sadie's surgery at Riverside. They already reached a deal with VitalGuard. I can get temporary privileges for the procedure. And after that…" He paused for effect. "I'll set up shop there permanently."

Another silence. Then, Stillson said coldly, "You are forgetting about your non-compete clause."

Liao smirked. "Then sue me. Happy to see you in court. You know there's been growing scrutiny and legislative efforts to limit or ban non-compete agreements, especially in health care. I'm willing to take the risk."

Another pause. Then a sigh. "And you're really willing to walk?"

"I am," Liao said. "And you know Riverside would be happy to have me."

Stillson inhaled sharply. "I'll…see what I can do."

Liao pressed. "You'll get this contract done now. Not just for Sadie—for everyone."

One last pause. Then, finally:

"I'll make some calls."

Liao hung up.

***

Two days later, VitalGuard and Wilkerson announced a new contract.

Sadie's surgery was scheduled within the week.

Liao never discovered exactly what transpired in those high-rise boardrooms. He only knew that the hospital caved when they realized they had more to lose than a single patient. As for VitalGuard, Liao was certain their shareholders were pleased with the outcome.

When he stepped into the OR to operate on Sadie, he felt something rare—victory.

Not just for her.

For everyone.

36. No Cure for Silence

A doctor believes in action as a remedy for censorship and erasure of critical medical knowledge.

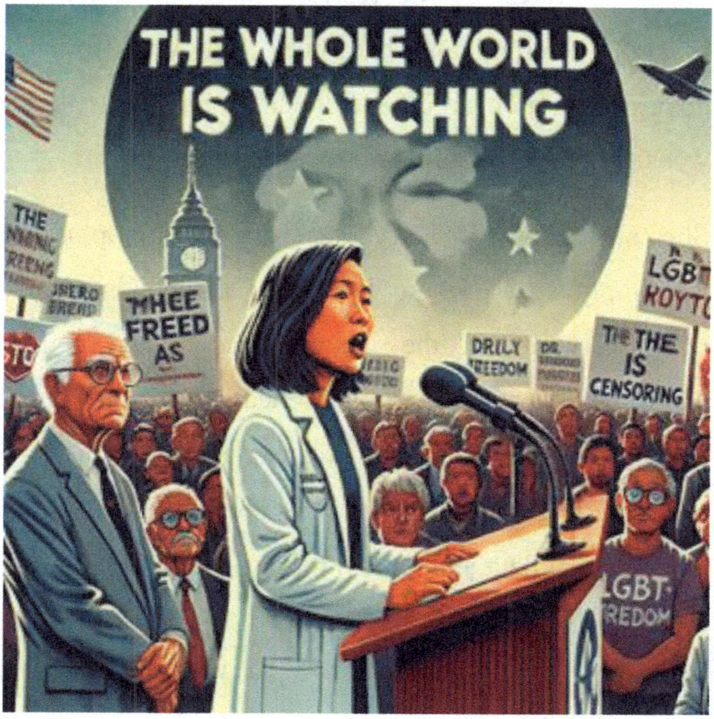

Dr. Lilly Nguyễn knew the risks of speaking out. She had spent her entire career navigating the delicate intersection of sociology, psychology, and medicine, advocating for the well-being of all patients, particularly those from marginalized communities. But nothing had prepared her for the full force of the government's suppression of her research.

It started with a phone call. A flat, bureaucratic voice informed her that her latest study, which detailed increased rates of depression in transgender and LGBTQ+ individuals, had been removed from the government-sponsored Healthcare Safety Alliance website. No explanation, no recourse. Just gone.

She sat in stunned silence, staring at her laptop screen, the empty space where her paper once existed. The research, years in the making, had linked gender-affirming care to improved health outcomes and emphasized the need for greater vigilance for those suffering from depression. It was solid science, backed by empirical data and patient narratives. But apparently, the wrong words had been used. "LGBTQ+," "gender identity," and "nonbinary" were now flagged as ideological threats.

Lilly's inbox flooded with emails from colleagues. Some were terrified; others were furious. "What's next?" one asked. "Are we moving from 'pray the gay away' to 'executive order the gay away'?" Another person wrote, "Next, researchers will probably not be able to use words like transformation, transactional, transposition, or the letters L B G T Q to designate anything. Imagine every EKG report being quashed because of 'QT'."

The new directive was clear. Government agencies were to "defend biological truth"—a phrase that sent a chill down her spine. The order's wording was vague enough to be wielded as a cudgel, excising not only her research but also any data that recognized LGBTQ+ individuals in healthcare discussions.

Lilly had spent her life fighting against systemic erasure. She wasn't about to stop now. She reached for her phone and dialed Dr. Kathy McGregor, a fellow researcher whose paper on anxiety disorders in transgender and nonbinary youths had also vanished overnight.

"We have to fight this," Lilly said, skipping pleasantries.

"I know," Kathy replied. "We're suing."

The lawsuit was a desperate attempt to claw back free speech, scientific integrity, and, most of all, the right of patients to receive accurate, inclusive medical care and safety information. Legal action was necessitated by the government's swift and ruthless policies. Government watchdogs had created a bogus surveillance agency—the

Bureau of Information Integrity (BII)—and declared that any mention of gender identities beyond the male-female binary was “misleading” and “contrary to national policy.” The bureau informed them that physicians do not possess an absolute right to publish their research on government websites.

Lilly knew what this meant. When powerful institutions controlled the narrative, medicine itself became a weapon. The chilling effect rippled through academia; researchers self-censored, avoiding “forbidden” words to protect their careers. Medical conferences removed panels on LGBTQ+ health. Funding for inclusive healthcare studies dried up. Entire populations were being written out of existence.

One night, as she was finalizing a speech for an underground network of healthcare professionals resisting the purge, she received an anonymous email. The subject line read, “They’re Watching.” The body contained a single sentence: “Be careful.”

She deleted the email but couldn’t shake the sense of dread. They wanted her afraid. They wanted her silent.

But Dr. Lilly Nguyễn had never been one to back down.

She took a deep breath and hit send on her latest article—this time, to an independent network of physicians and journalists. If the government did not house the truth, then the people would. The fight was far from over.

***

Lilly sat across from Dr. Robert Howell in a tiny café near the courthouse. The air smelled of burnt coffee and tension. Howell had been a mentor in residency, a baby boomer with an encyclopedic knowledge of rock music and an unexpected obsession with The Doors.

"You know what Jim Morrison said," Howell began, stirring his espresso. "'You cannot petition the Lord with prayer.'"

Lilly smirked. "And yet here we are, petitioning the courts."

Howell smiled. "Prayer might bring comfort, but it won't change policy. You need strategy, not faith." He leaned in. "They expect you to roll over."

"They want us afraid," Lilly admitted. "Afraid of losing funding, losing our licenses, losing the ability to help patients who don't look like them, act like them, think like them, or speak like them."

Howell nodded. “And that’s exactly why you can’t back down. Do you remember what I told you about the ‘68 convention?”

“The whole world is watching,” Lilly said, almost to herself. She could still hear his voice from years ago, describing the scene in Chicago—the cops, the blood, the protestors chanting as the nation watched in horror. “That’s what we need. To make them watch.”

Howell’s eyes lit up. “Exactly. You need to make noise. Get the medical journals involved; get international eyes on this. This isn’t just about your paper. It’s about the precedent.”

Lilly exhaled. “They’ve already started silencing others. If we don’t fight this now, what’s next? They’ll erase every mention of transgender health. They’ll take out LGBTQ+ specialists from insurance networks. It’s systematic erasure.”

Howell’s face hardened. “Which means you have to go public. Bigger than just the lawsuit. The media, rallies, and testimony before Congress. You have to make them listen, even if they don’t want to.”

Lilly hesitated. “What if I lose everything?”

Howell smirked. "Bob Dylan said it best: 'When you ain't got nothing, you got nothing to lose.' You're already fighting with everything on the line, so you may as well go all in. They don't fear the lawsuit. They fear you. You're a doctor, not a politician. You speak the truth, and they can't afford that."

There was a pregnant pause between them. Then Lilly pulled out her phone and sent a text to Kathy. 'We're going public. Full press. The whole world is watching.'

Howell grinned. "Now that's the fighter I trained," while managing to borrow one more lyric, this time from Don Henley and The Eagles: "We haven't had that spirit here since 1969."

37. Unmatched

A medical student's determination pays off after receiving heartbreaking news.

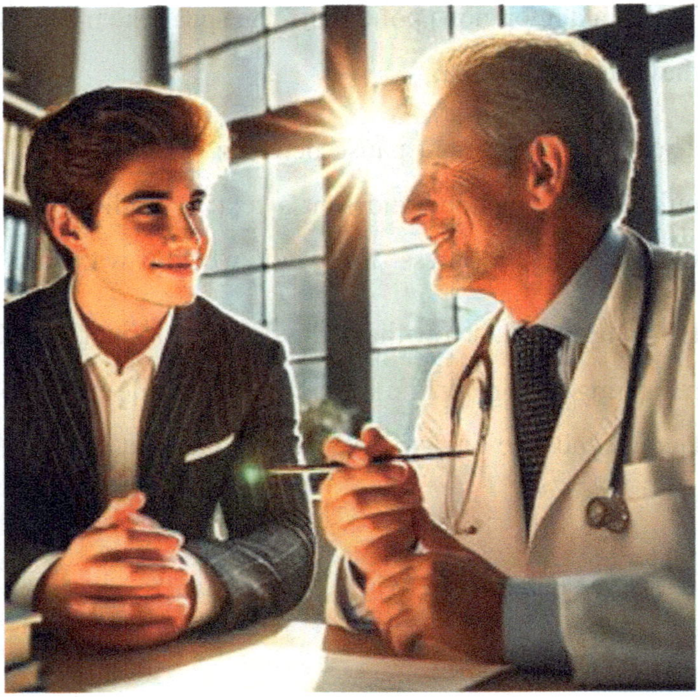

The knock on the office door was hesitant, almost reluctant.

“Come in,” Dr. Ted Haskins called, setting aside the research article he had been reading.

The door creaked open, revealing Dr. Logan Davenport, shoulders slumped, eyes hollow. He stepped inside, closed the door softly, then stood there, as if the weight of the world pinned him in place.

"I take it the news wasn't what you were expecting," Haskins said, gesturing toward the chair across from his desk.

Logan sank into it. "There is no news. I didn't match." His voice was quiet and flat. "Dermatology. Not a single program. I don't understand. My scores were stellar, my letters—unbelievable. The interviewers loved me. And yet—nothing."

Haskins leaned forward, hands clasped. "Logan, I won't deny it. That's a gut punch. I can only imagine how you're feeling."

Logan gave a hollow chuckle. "Can you? Because right now, I feel like the universe just told me I'm not good enough."

Haskins sighed. "I get it. You spent years crafting the perfect application, checking every box, and still…"

Logan clenched his jaw. "I don't know what I did wrong."

"Maybe nothing. Maybe it was a numbers game. Maybe there were faculty politics at play. Maybe the algorithm that runs the Match just flipped a coin in the wrong direction."

"None of that makes me feel better."

"I know." Haskins let the silence settle. "What's your next step?"

"I don't know. I mean, there's the Supplemental Offer and Acceptance Program—SOAP—but most of the open spots aren't in dermatology. If I go that route, I might have to pivot specialties entirely. But the thought of giving up on derm? It makes me sick."

Haskins nodded. "So, you have options. You can enter SOAP and find a residency, even if it's not your first choice. You can take a gap year, do research and strengthen your application, and reapply next cycle. Or—"

"Or I give up and call it quits," Logan finished bitterly.

Haskins frowned. "That's not what I was going to say. I was going to say you could take a step back and reassess why you chose dermatology in the first place. Was it prestige? Income? Lifestyle? Or was it something deeper?"

Logan was silent for a long moment. "It was all of the above. I love the mix of procedural and clinical observation, even the pathology. And yeah, I won't lie—a predictable schedule and solid compensation were part of it."

Haskins nodded. "Those are valid reasons. But let me ask you this: Is your love for medicine tied solely to dermatology? If I told you that next year you'd match into family medicine or psychiatry or emergency medicine, would you still feel fulfilled?"

Logan exhaled sharply. "I don't know. Right now, it feels like everything's been ripped away."

Haskins tapped his desk. "Then take the time to grieve. You lost something today—an expectation, a dream on a timeline you thought was set in stone. But this isn't the end of the story. It's just a plot twist."

Logan ran a hand through his hair. "It's hard to see that right now. Everyone else is celebrating. I just want to disappear."

"I get that. But listen, Logan. How you handle this moment—the resilience you build—will define you far more than the specialty you end up in. The best doctors aren't just the ones who match straight away. They're the ones who learn how to manage setbacks with grace."

Logan swallowed hard. "So, what do I do now?"

Haskins leaned back. "You take the weekend. Feel everything you need to feel. Then on Monday, we strategize. We find a way forward. Because you, Logan Davenport, are still going to be a damn good doctor. Match or no match?"

After the conversation faded, Logan mustered the faintest of smiles for the first time that day.

***

A year had passed since that fateful day, and Logan found himself once again standing outside Dr. Haskins' office. This time, his knock was firm, resonating with a newfound determination.

"Come in," Haskins called from within.

Logan entered, his demeanor a blend of pride and exhaustion. "I did it. I matched—dermatology."

Haskins' face lit up with genuine delight. "Logan, that's fantastic news! Sit down and tell me everything."

Taking a seat, Logan exhaled deeply. "After our conversation last year, I took your advice to heart. I dedicated myself to strengthening my application. I secured a research position at a leading dermatology department, immersing myself in projects that led to two poster presentations and future publications. I attended national conferences, networked extensively, and sought mentorship from respected figures in the field. I also revised my personal statement, ensuring it truly reflected my passion and growth over the past year."

Haskins nodded appreciatively. "Your perseverance is commendable. It's worth noting that dermatology is one of the most competitive specialties. I think that in recent years only about three-fourths of applicants to dermatology residency programs successfully matched. That's quite an impressive feat on your part!"

Logan acknowledged the statistic with a somber nod. "I was aware of the odds. It made me question my path at times, but I couldn't see myself in any other specialty."

"Understandable," Haskins replied. "You know some of the things we talked about last year — doing research and obtaining letters of recommendation from dermatologists — can definitely enhance your chances the second time around. It seems you strategically addressed these areas."

"Exactly," Logan agreed. "I also made sure to build strong relationships during my rotations and sought feedback to continually improve. It was a challenging year, but every effort was worth it."

Haskins leaned back, a look of pride evident in his eyes. "Logan, your journey exemplifies tenacity and dedication. You've not only achieved your goal but also grown immensely as a professional. The field of dermatology will be better with you in it."

A genuine smile spread across Logan's face. "Thank you, Dr. Haskins. Your support and guidance were instrumental in this journey."

"Remember," Haskins added, "this experience has equipped you with a deep empathy for future colleagues and patients facing setbacks. It's a valuable perspective that will serve you well in your career."

Logan nodded thoughtfully. "I hadn't considered that, but you're right. This journey has taught me the importance of perseverance and compassion."

"Now," Haskins said, standing up and extending his hand, "go celebrate this well-deserved achievement. You've earned it."

Logan shook his mentor's hand firmly, gratitude shining in his eyes. "I will. And thank you, truly, for everything."

As he left the office, Logan felt a profound sense of accomplishment. The road had been arduous, but it had led him to where he was meant to be—a future dermatologist ready to make a difference.

38. Dedicated

A physician is *rewarded* for his immeasurable impact on students.

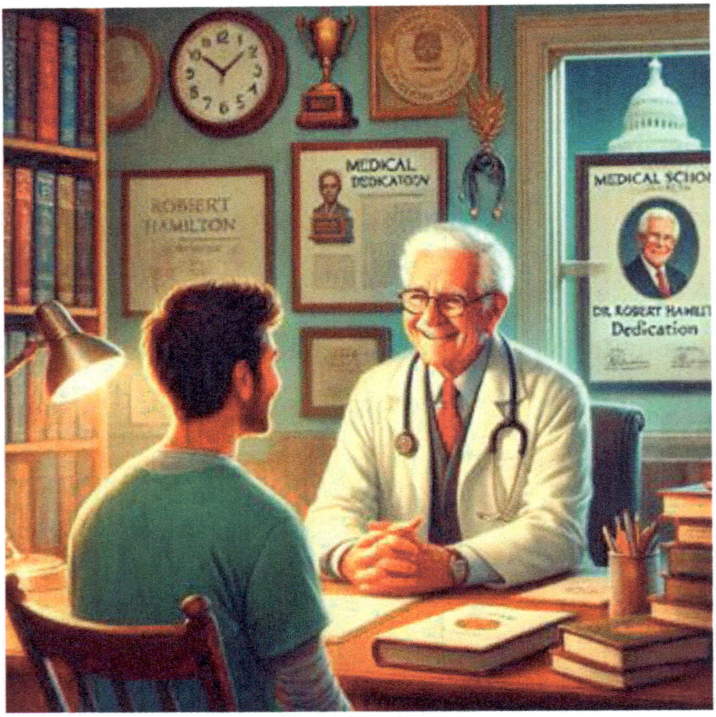

Dr. Robert "Bob" Hamilton never cared much for awards. Oh, they were nice, he supposed. He had plenty of them—plaques, framed certificates, golden apples, and various accolades that medical institutions had handed him over the years. They lined the walls of his modest office in the teaching hospital, gathering dust while he remained far more interested in the living, breathing individuals who walked through his door.

"Dr. Hamilton, do you have a moment?" A nervous young voice asked from his doorway. It was Nate Reynolds, a fourth-year medical student who had just finished his final rounds under Dr. Hamilton's watch.

"For you, Nate? Always. Come in. Sit. You look like you have something on your mind."

Nate hesitated before settling into the chair opposite Dr. Hamilton's desk. "It's just—well, I wanted to thank you. For everything. I was struggling this year, really wondering if I had what it takes, and you...you saw something in me when I couldn't see it in myself."

Dr. Hamilton leaned back, his ever-present kind smile appearing. "Ah, Nate, don't thank me. Thank yourself for sticking with it. Medicine isn't just about brilliance; it's about resilience. You proved that every day."

Nate nodded, but his hands were still clasped tightly in his lap. "Sir, I also wanted to tell you… The class is dedicating our yearbook to you. They asked me to deliver the good news because they were aware of our special relationship."

For the first time in a long time, Dr. Hamilton found himself momentarily speechless.

"Me?" he finally said, astonished. "Why me?"

"Because you embody what it means to be dedicated," Nate said earnestly. "Not just to medicine, but to us. To teaching. To mentorship. I mean, every student here has a 'Dr. Hamilton story.' Like how you stayed late to go over cases with Maggie when she was struggling in internal medicine. Or how you sat with Diego in the cafeteria after his first patient died and made sure he was okay. You taught us more than medicine—you taught us how to be doctors."

Dr. Hamilton exhaled slowly, his heart unexpectedly full. He thought of the late nights and the countless hours spent explaining, guiding, and listening. It had never felt like a sacrifice. It had been the only way he knew how to live.

Nate's eyes brightened as he added, "And honestly, we should've known from the very beginning. I still remember orientation. We were all terrified, sitting there as different departments listed off assigned readings and impossible expectations. I thought I had made the biggest mistake of my life coming to med school. Then you walked in. You cracked jokes about 'the grind,' 'the jock,' and 'the one-upsman'—how we should leave those stereotypes behind—and suddenly, we could all breathe again. And when you told us that there was no secret system designed to weed us out, that we all belonged here—that changed everything. You gave us hope before we even knew we needed it."

Dr. Hamilton was amazed, shaking his head. "That was a long time ago, but I remember that day well. I saw a sea of nervous faces, and I knew you all needed reassurance more than another lecture on coursework. You did all belong here—you just didn't know it yet."

Nate smiled, then hesitated before adding, "You know, I realized over time that your dedication wasn't just about medicine. It extended beyond the hospital. I remember the time I ran into you and your wife at the community fundraiser. It was the first time I saw you outside of your white coat. You weren't just 'Dr. Hamilton'—you were a husband, a father, a person who gave just as much to his family as he did to his students and patients. It made me realize that being dedicated doesn't mean sacrificing everything else—it means bringing the same passion to every part of your life."

At home, Dr. Hamilton's dedication had been matched step for step by his wife, Vicki, a devoted therapist whose quiet wisdom had guided countless patients through their darkest times. She had understood, better than anyone, what it meant to give oneself fully to others. Over the years, she had been his rock, his confidante—even his tennis partner—and often the one to remind him when it was time to step away from work and be present with their family.

Their children, Michael and Andrea, had grown up in a household where medicine was not just a career but a calling. Both had followed in their parents' footsteps, Michael as a surgeon and Andrea as a pediatrician. "We never stood a chance," Andrea often joked at family gatherings. "With parents like you two, how could we do anything else?"

As Nate left, Dr. Hamilton turned to his cluttered desk, his fingers brushing against an old, worn stethoscope. The weight of the years pressed upon him, but so did something else—gratitude.

He had given medicine everything he had. But he had never done it alone.

And somehow, it had given him even more in return.

39. Overcoming the Chore of Medicine

Two physicians discuss how to innovate and focus on medicine's core, not chores.

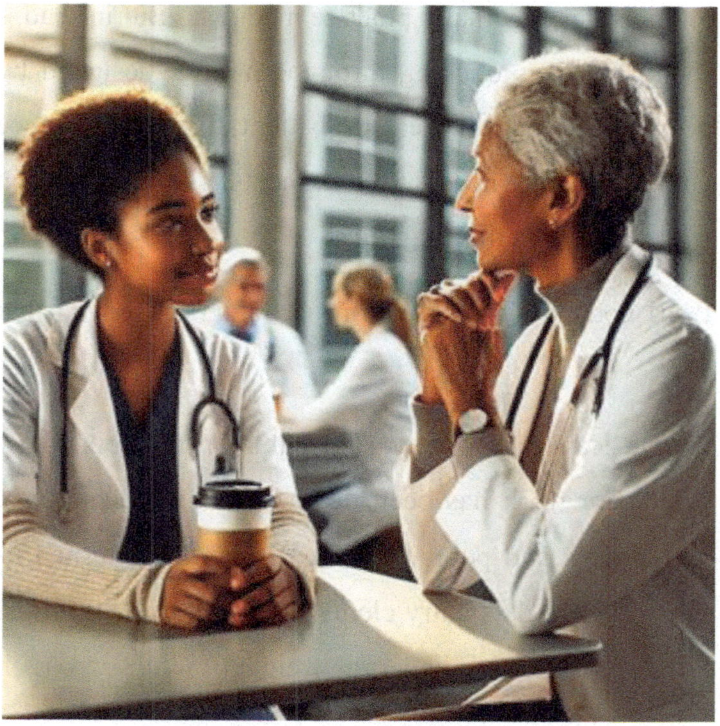

Dr. Amina Nyota clenched her cup of coffee, her mind heavy with frustration typical of early-career physicians. Across from her, Dr. Pearl Baker, wiser than her years, watched with quiet patience.

"Pearl," Amina finally said, exhaling, "I don't think I can do this anymore."

Pearl was uncertain what "this" meant. "This job?"

"This system." Amina glanced around the bustling hospital cafeteria. "I went into medicine to help people—to innovate, to actually practice medicine. But instead, I spend my days clicking through an EHR designed by people who've never treated a patient, fighting insurance companies over necessary treatments, and drowning in endless, useless meetings."

Pearl nodded slowly. "You're not alone in feeling that way."

Amina leaned forward. "I read this article about how healthcare work has been degraded—how technology, regulations, and poor workflow design have turned us into glorified data entry clerks instead of doctors. I feel like I'm suffocating under the weight of it all."

"I hear you. But let me ask—do you want to leave medicine, or just this version of it?"

Amina hesitated, then sighed. "I don't know. I used to love this job. Now, I dread coming in. It's not just the workload. It's everything."

Pearl leaned back, studying her. "Tell me more."

Amina glanced away. "I feel stuck. Like I'm not learning anything new. My ideas don't seem to matter. And honestly? I don't even feel like I'm making a difference. My skills feel wasted on bureaucratic nonsense."

Pearl nodded. "That's a lot. And it makes sense you'd feel disillusioned. Have you thought about what exactly is making you want to walk away? Because leaving medicine is a big decision—it's not just about quitting a job."

Amina exhaled. "I've thought about it. I don't think it's one thing. It's—" she counted off on her fingers. "I feel like I've stopped growing. The stress is constant. I don't feel heard. And worst of all? I feel like I'm losing my passion."

Pearl watched her, then said gently, "That's a dangerous place to be."

Amina gave a humorless chuckle. "Tell me about it."

Pearl tapped her fingers on the table. "So, let's break it down. You're clearly unhappy, but quitting without a plan might just swap one problem for another. Have you thought about changing settings instead of careers? Maybe private practice, academia, or even consulting?"

Amina bit her lip. "I've thought about it, but would it be any different? Medicine everywhere seems broken."

Pearl smiled wryly. "It is. But not equally. Some places do it better. And some physicians carve out roles that allow them to focus on what they love. Have you looked at options that align with what you actually want?"

Amina shook her head. "I've been too caught up in the frustration to even think about that."

Pearl leaned in. "Then let's start there. What excites you about medicine, even now?"

Amina was quiet for a moment. "Patient care. Teaching. Cutting-edge treatments. But none of that feels possible anymore."

Pearl's gaze was steady. "It can be. If you design your career instead of letting it be designed for you."

Amina exhaled. "So, you're saying don't make an impulsive decision."

"I'm saying make an informed one," Pearl corrected. "Leaving might be the right call. But first, ask yourself, is it the job? The institution? The system? Or is it something you can change?"

Amina was quiet, absorbing the words. Finally, she nodded. "I need to think."

Pearl smiled. "Good. And when you're ready, let's talk about what's next."

For the first time in a long time, Amina felt something other than pessimism—she felt possibility.

***

Several weeks later, Amina and Pearl met again for lunch. Amina felt ready, determined. Her mind was clearer.

"I think I know what I need to do, Pearl," Amina said, her voice steadier than before. "I don't want to leave medicine. I want to take back control of my career. I want to be my own boss, in the way that actually matters."

Pearl nodded. "Good. Now let's define exactly what that looks like for you."

Amina exhaled. "I want out of this grind—the administrative nonsense, the productivity quotas, the feeling that I'm just a cog in the machine. But I still love teaching. I love mentoring. I miss the intellectual challenge of real medicine."

Pearl smiled. "Sounds like an academic career might be the right move."

Amina hesitated. "I've thought about it, but…the salary cut worries me. I have loans. Responsibilities."

"It's a valid concern," Pearl admitted. "Academic medicine typically pays less than private practice or hospital-employed positions. But in exchange, you get a different kind of currency—time, intellectual fulfillment, and mentorship opportunities. You'll be shaping the next generation of physicians. And if you play your cards right, you can carve out research or leadership roles that supplement your income."

Amina nodded, absorbing the trade-offs. Then Pearl's expression shifted slightly.

"But there's something else I need to be real with you about," she said. "The glass ceiling."

Amina looked puzzled. "Meaning?"

"Meaning academic medicine still has its barriers, especially for women, and especially for women of color," Pearl said plainly. "It's improving, but we both know that leadership roles, high-impact research opportunities, and tenure tracks don't always come as easily for us as they do for others."

Amina sighed. "Yeah, I know the stats. Fewer Black women in leadership, fewer grants awarded, and more bias in evaluations."

"No question," Pearl said. "I'm not saying don't do it—far from it. But go in with your eyes open. Find mentors who will advocate for you. Be intentional about how you seek promotions and research funding. And, most importantly, document everything—your achievements, your leadership, and your teaching. Don't assume people will just notice. Make them notice."

Amina nodded slowly. "So…I'll have to work twice as hard."

Pearl gave her a knowing look. "Hasn't that always been the case?"

Amina let out a small laugh. "Fair point." She took a deep breath. "Okay. I can do this. But how do I start?"

Pearl leaned in. "First, make yourself visible. Reach out to your old professors, attendings, and anyone in academia who remembers your work. Networking isn't just about who you know—it's about who knows you. Next, check job boards, university career sites, and medical journals. Even cold-email department chairs if you see an opportunity that fits."

"Got it," Amina said. "And my CV?"

"Polish it," Pearl advised. "Highlight your teaching experience, your research, and your leadership. Make it clear why you're the perfect fit for an academic role. And one more thing—don't wait until you resign. Start planting the seeds now. You don't want a gap in your career if you can avoid it."

Amina checked her watch—lunch was over. But instead of feeling drained, she felt fueled. She stood, rolling her shoulders back.

"You know," she said, a small smile playing at her lips, "I've been feeling stuck for months. But now? Now, I feel like I have a way forward."

Pearl grinned. "Because you do. You're taking control. No more waiting for medicine to fix itself—you're designing your own path. Act like you're the CEO of your own company—report to your 'board of mentors,' and let your core competencies report to you."

Amina met her gaze with self-determination. "Wow! What great advice! Thanks, Pearl. I needed this."

"Anytime," Pearl said, standing. "Now go get that job."

As Amina walked out of the cafeteria and back into the maze of hospital hallways, the fluorescent lights didn't seem quite so harsh. She could honestly say she wasn't dreading what came next—she was planning for it.

40. The Rise and Fall of Faisal Ali

Doctors realized too late that *this* "Ali" was not the greatest.

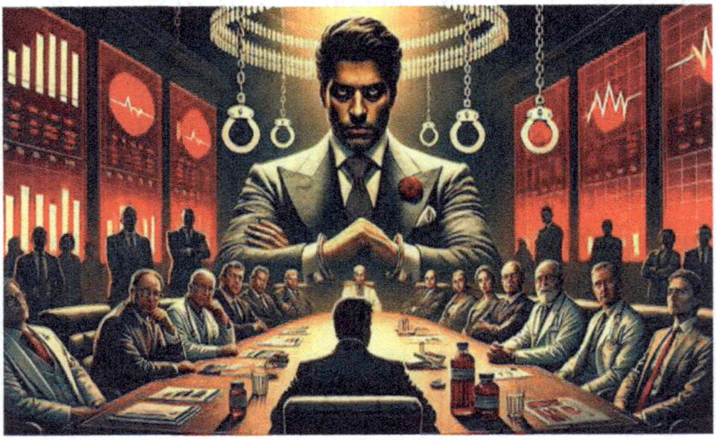

Faisal Ali sat at the head of the long conference table, his fingers steepled under his chin. He scanned the room, his dark eyes locking onto the physicians before him, all department chairs, each squirming uncomfortably in their seats.

"Let me be clear," Ali said, his voice cold and measured. "You will not cross me. Those who do will live to regret it."

A murmur rippled through the crowd, quickly silenced by the weight of his words. He had made his position known. This was not a negotiation. It was a decree.

Ali had started as a procurement officer, handling contracts for medical supplies. But he was hungry for more. Within a decade, he maneuvered his way through the ranks, becoming CFO, then COO, and finally, the CEO of HealthSpan Hospitals. His rise was meteoric and not marked by innovation or compassion but by a relentless pursuit of power, an uncanny ability to manipulate board members, and a ruthless elimination of anyone who dared to oppose him.

At first, his vision seemed compelling. He spoke of transformation, of an integrated healthcare system that would rival the largest in the nation, spurred by the acquisition of community practices and hospitals. The board, dazzled by his confidence, handed him unchecked authority. Expansion followed at breakneck speed—not only were hospitals and practices acquired, but medical schools and residency programs were folded into the enterprise, an empire built on a foundation of debt.

Behind closed doors, Ali ruled by fear. Executives who failed to meet financial targets were publicly humiliated in meetings. “You think you can run this place better?” he once barked at a COO who dared question his aggressive spending. “Good luck finding another job in this industry.” He was fired on the spot.

The CFO, a once-respected financial expert, found himself reduced to a glorified accountant. “The numbers don’t add up,” he whispered to a colleague after one particularly difficult meeting. “He’s shifting funds between hospitals like a shell game. This isn’t sustainable.”

But no one dared challenge Ali. Not the doctors, who feared retaliation. Not the executives, who watched their predecessors cast out in disgrace. Not even the board, now filled with his handpicked loyalists.

The first sign of trouble came when payroll was delayed for the first time in the company’s history. Then came whispers of unpaid vendors, halted construction projects, and financial reports that no longer made sense.

An emergency board meeting was called. Ali, still exuding confidence, brushed off concerns. “Temporary cash flow issues,” he declared. “Nothing we can’t manage.”

But the truth was far more dire—and sinister. HealthSpan was losing nearly a million dollars a day. Yet, as the organization was hemorrhaging money, Ali continued to pay himself and his cronies lavishly. He lived in a mansion supplied by the organization. Five of HealthSpan's top executives were in the top 10 best-paid hospital executives in the city.

Eventually it was discovered that funds had been siphoned from solvent hospitals to prop up failing acquisitions. Money from endowed chairs was used for operations. Federal investigators began sniffing around, tipped off by discrepancies in tax filings.

***

Dr. Clara Voeller sat alone in HealthSpan's bustling cafeteria, her tray untouched. Around her, colleagues murmured in hushed tones, their voices a blend of anxiety and disbelief. Rumors of HealthSpan's impending closure had spread like wildfire.

"Did you hear?" Dr. Gabriel ("Gabe") Ramos, a seasoned cardiologist, slid into the seat across from her. "They're saying we might not even get severance."

Clara sighed, pushing her salad around her plate. "I heard. It's like the rug's been pulled out from under us. I mean, just last week they were talking about expansion. Now they're talking bankruptcy."

Gabe shook his head, his expression a mix of frustration and resignation. "Expansion? More like implosion. I can't believe they didn't see this coming."

"Or maybe they did and just didn't care," Clara replied, her voice tinged with bitterness. "What about your patients?"

Gabe stared away for a moment. "I'm trying to figure out who I might need to transfer to other practices—the critical ones and those in the middle of treatment—but it's a nightmare."

"You want to talk about a nightmare?" Clara responded, becoming emotional. "What about the residents? They'll have to scramble to find new placements! Who's going to accept them in the middle of the year? Think how they'll be uprooted. New cities. New programs—likely second tier. And their poor families—so much disruption to their partners and kids."

Across the room, Dr. Valentina Lopez, a pediatrician known for her unwavering optimism, approached their table. “Hey, have you guys found any leads on new positions?” she asked, her voice carrying a forced cheerfulness.

Clara shook her head. “I've sent out a few applications in anticipation something like this might happen, but it’s tough—and there’s been no official announcement. The market’s saturated with all of us looking at the same time.”

Valentina nodded, her smile faltering. “I know. I have a couple of interviews lined up, but who knows if they’ll pan out? I should have trusted my instincts and started searching months ago. What’s that famous line: ‘You don’t have to be a weatherman to know which way the wind blows.’ I guess I failed at forecasting!”

Gabe leaned forward, lowering his voice. “You know, I heard some of the execs are already lining up jobs at other big systems. It’s like they just walked away from this mess.”

Clara’s eyes narrowed. “Of course they are. They get to move on while we clean up the aftermath.”

As the three doctors sat in silence, the enormity of their situation settled over them. HealthSpan had been more than just a job; it was a community, a place where they had built careers and friendships. A teaching hospital, where some trainees stayed on and the doctors who taught them were able to see firsthand the fruits of their labors. All that is possibly gone now.

"Do you remember the gala last year? Valentina said suddenly, breaking the silence. "They promised us a future full of innovation and growth. It feels like a bad joke now."

Gabe nodded. "Yeah, and to think we were all so excited. We swallowed the Kool-Aid. It's hard to believe it might be the end."

Clara leaned in, her voice resolute. "We can't let this define us. We've built something here, even if HealthSpan couldn't hold it together. We owe it to our patients—and to ourselves—to find a way forward."

Valentina smiled, some of her optimism returning. "You're right. We've got the skills and the passion. We'll land on our feet."

She was the eternal optimist.

***

When the news finally broke, it was catastrophic. HealthSpan filed for bankruptcy—one of the largest nonprofit health system bankruptcies in U.S. history. Thousands lost their jobs. Hospitals shuttered overnight. Patients were left scrambling for care. Attendings and residents searched for open positions. Some doctors were absorbed by local institutions, but many were displaced or left hanging in the balance.

The regional healthcare landscape was changed forever.

Ali was nowhere to be found.

The FBI tracked him to a luxury villa in the Caribbean. When they finally brought him back in handcuffs, he still smirked for the cameras. "This is all politics," he sneered. "They needed a scapegoat."

In court, the evidence was overwhelming—fraudulent financial reports and kickbacks disguised as consulting fees. Endowed funds illegally raided. Ali's inner circle crumbled, one executive after another turning against him in exchange for lighter sentences.

In the end, Faisal Ali, once hailed as a visionary, was charged with multiple felonies, striking a plea bargain to serve time in the county jail for the misuse of charitable funds. His empire lay in ruins, a cautionary tale of unchecked ambition, fear-driven leadership, and the consequences of allowing one man to wield absolute power.

As he was led away in an orange jumpsuit, a former physician from HealthSpan pointed a finger and shouted, “You warned us not to cross you. Turns out, you were the one who crossed the line.”

41. The Measured Leader

A doctor's effective leadership requires emotional intelligence—and an understanding of the "80/20 rule."

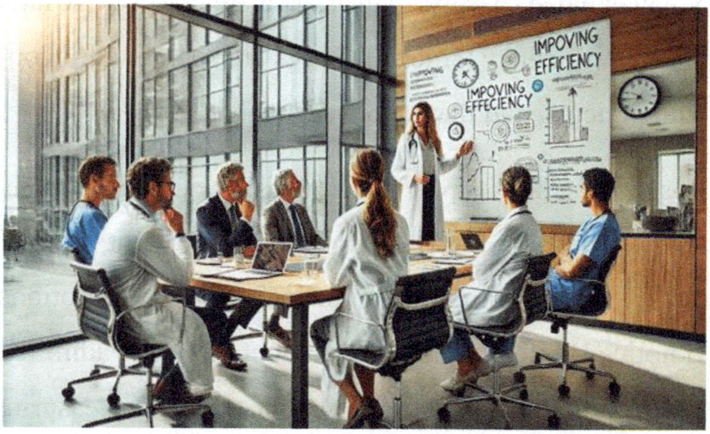

Dr. Rose Whitman, Chief Wellness Officer at Summit Health System, sat at the head of the conference table, her fingers lightly drumming against the polished wood. Across from her, Dr. Nolan Bainbridge, the hospital's CMO, leaned back in his chair, chin propped up by his arm and hand. The tension in the room was palpable, certainly not a reflection of the committee's name: The Wellness Committee.

"I've been thinking about our situation," Rose began, planting both feet firmly on the ground, steadying herself. "There's been a lot of friction between the administration and the medical staff. I want to understand your perspective first."

Nolan exhaled sharply. "The issue is time, Rose. We have to meet efficiency targets. Doctors are spending too long with patients, and that's not sustainable."

Rose took a slow sip of water, pausing deliberately. She felt a flicker of irritation rise but caught herself, recognizing the importance of managing her emotions. "I notice I'm feeling frustrated about this," she admitted. "We're measuring efficiency, but are we measuring impact?"

Nolan grimaced. "Impact?"

She nodded. "Let's explore what success looks like for both of us. If we push physicians to see more patients per hour, are we truly improving care?" She drew a quick timeline on the whiteboard before her. "What happens six months down the line? More readmissions? Lower patient satisfaction? Burnout? That's not good for anyone."

Nolan tapped a pen against the table. "You have a point. But the hospital board doesn't see it that way."

Rose leaned in slightly. "I appreciate you bringing this to my attention. And I want to ensure I understand correctly—are you saying the board values speed over quality?"

Nolan hesitated. "Not in so many words. But they see numbers. And the numbers say shorter visits equal higher throughput."

Rose let the silence settle for a moment. She reminded herself that leadership wasn't about winning an argument—it was about guiding a conversation. She bit her lip, and instead of blurting out, 'This isn't a McDonald's drive-through,' she retained her composure and reflected. "Can we pause here? I want to process this fully." She glanced at the other physicians in the room, their eyes fixed on her. "Let's focus on solutions we can both support."

Dr. Connie Ramirez, an infectious disease specialist, spoke up. "What if we find the 20% of inefficiencies causing 80% of delays? Maybe it's redundant paperwork, excessive prior authorizations, or our cumbersome EHR system?"

Nolan rubbed his chin. "That…could work."

Rose turned slightly sideways, diffusing the tension. "What feels most important to address first?"

Nolan sighed. "Physician burnout. If we lose good doctors, none of this matters."

Rose nodded. "I see this differently, but I'm curious about your view. Is it burnout from patient care or from the administrative hassles and bottlenecks that slow down patient care and burden physicians without adding real value?"

"Both," Nolan admitted. "But mostly bureaucracy."

Connie grinned. "So, let's optimize. The 80/20 rule applies here, too. If 80% of paperwork is just for compliance, but only 20% truly impacts patient care, let's cut the fluff."

Nolan exhaled. "Alright. Let's do it. But we need a plan."

Rose smiled, feeling the weight of leadership settle on her shoulders—not as a burden, but as a responsibility.

"I commit to presenting a proposal by next week. Can we set a follow-up?"

Nolan pulled out his phone. "Blocking off time now."

As the meeting wrapped up, Rose looked around. "Thank you for having this conversation. This is good teamwork—not just for our institution, but for our patients."

Nolan chuckled. "And for our sanity."

Connie winked, remarking, "Let's prove Woody Allen was right when he said, '80% of success is just showing up.'"

***

The committee reconvened the following week in the same conference room, the whiteboard now adorned with scribbled notes from last week's session. The attendees were more than a little bleary-eyed, but the energy in the room was positive, a mixture of curiosity and determination to figure out how to simplify their complex world.

Rose, always quick to find humor in any situation, leaned against the podium with a grin, glancing around the room. “Well, folks, it looks like about 80% of you showed up from last week, and that, my friends, constitutes a quorum!” She laughed at the groans and tired chuckles in response, her smile infectious as the group settled in.

“Okay, let’s dive right in,” she said, getting straight to the heart of the matter. “Last week we laid the groundwork, and this week I want to take a deeper dive into the 80/20 rule. We talked about reducing, modifying, or eliminating certain operations or requirements that drain time and resources, and today we’re going to see how we can really apply that.”

She clicked the remote, and a new slide popped up on the screen with the bold heading: The 80/20 Rule: Efficiency Through Focus. Beneath it were bullet points summarizing key topics from last week's meeting. She pointed to the first item.

“Now, some of you raised great points last week, and I want us to think critically about this. Let's look at the processes, tasks, or services that make up 80% of our time but contribute only 20% to our overall success. What can we adjust, streamline, or get rid of altogether?”

John, a new member of the committee, cleared his throat. "Well, one thing that stands out to me immediately is our current reporting system. We spend hours pulling data from different sources, cleaning it up, and formatting it for the monthly board meeting. It's exhausting, and yet, if we're honest, most of the board members only glance at it before moving on."

Rose nodded thoughtfully. "Great point. Is there any way we could automate some of that, or at least make the reports less detailed without losing the essential information?"

Latoya, the head of operations, chimed in. "We could definitely use a software tool to aggregate the data. Maybe we can even present it in a dashboard format so they can focus on key metrics and trends. That would cut down on the manual work and give them what they need at a glance."

"Exactly," Rose said. "And the 80/20 rule applies here, too. If 80% of the report's details don't contribute to decision-making, let's stop spending so much time on them."

The group nodded in agreement, jotting down notes. Rose moved to the next point on the slide.

“Another area we could apply this is in meetings. We all know how easily meetings can eat up a disproportionate amount of time. I’ve been tracking some of our recent ones, and I noticed that only 20% of our discussions are really driving the decisions forward. The rest...well, they feel more like a collection of side conversations and grievances.”

Everyone shifted uncomfortably, but they knew it was true.

John raised an eyebrow. “Are you suggesting we eliminate meetings altogether?”

“Not necessarily,” Rose said with a smile. “But we could be more strategic. Let’s consider shortening meeting durations, sticking to strict agendas and start times, and limiting attendance to the people who absolutely need to be there. We might find that some meetings could be cut down to just 20 minutes or even eliminated entirely.”

“That’s going to be a hard sell,” Latoya said, half-laughing. “But I see your point.”

"Exactly," Rose replied. "It's not about eliminating all meetings—it's about being intentional with our time. Let's aim for quality, not quantity."

They spent the next hour dissecting more areas that could benefit from the 80/20 rule. Some of the suggestions included streamlining the onboarding process for new hires, delegating redundant documentation requirements, and reconsidering the frequency of certain administrative tasks.

By the end of the meeting, the group had outlined several key areas where they could implement changes. Rose felt optimistic. "I'm not suggesting we can change everything overnight, but if we start small and prioritize, we'll begin to see meaningful improvements in efficiency."

As they wrapped up, John leaned back in his chair, a thoughtful expression on his face. "You know, Rose, you might be onto something. If we can focus on the 20% that actually drives results, we might just free up enough time to make real progress."

Rose grinned. "That's the idea! And maybe we'll all get a little more time back in our lives." She looked at him playfully. “And who knows? Perhaps next week, we’ll have a full 100% turnout.”

The group laughed, their energy renewed as they filed out of the room, eager to start tackling the changes that were now firmly on the horizon.

42. The Silent Letter

A physician's adage, "See one, do one, teach one," reverberates in the surgical suite.

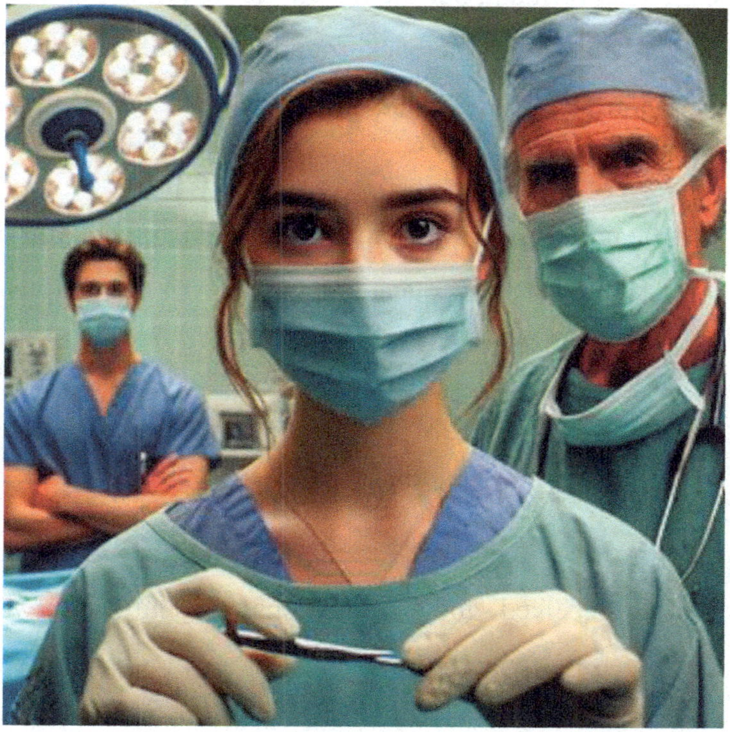

Lucy Knapp dreaded the email. The moment her schedule for third-year rotations arrived, her heart pounded as she scrolled past internal medicine and pediatrics, hoping, praying—

Surgery.

Her stomach dropped.

Weeks before the rotation started, anxiety gnawed at her. She didn't belong in an OR. She could barely introduce herself to patients without stammering. Her classmates called her brilliant, but she feared she was an imposter, a shadow lurking in the background. She joked that even her name, "Nap," reflected her nature. "The 'K' is silent. Like me."

But there was nothing silent about the man who would oversee her surgical education.

Dr. Jackson Harding, a seasoned general surgeon with a reputation for demanding excellence, wasted no time assessing his newest trainee.

"You're Lucy Knapp," he said, scanning his list. "I see you've received good evaluations in your first two rotations. But you don't talk much. You know, medicine and peds are more cerebral than surgery. Those attendings are more likely to accommodate your personality. Well, that'll change here."

Lucy swallowed.

"Surgery isn't for spectators. You'll follow SODOTO: See one, do one, teach one. Ever heard of it?"

She nodded hesitantly, heart hammering. “I've heard of it, but I’m not sure I really understand how it works.”

“Good,” he said. “You’ll find out. Now, let’s get to work.”

The first case was a routine appendectomy. Lucy stood behind Dr. Harding, watching as he navigated the anatomy with a mastery that made everything look simple. Too simple.

“See one,” he murmured as he worked.

Afterward, he turned to her. “Next time, you’ll do it.”

She barely slept that night. Surely, he hadn’t meant she’d actually perform a surgery. She was just a student—wasn’t she supposed to spend most of the time retracting and suctioning, not cutting?

A week went by before Lucy had the chance to scrub in on another appendectomy. Meanwhile, she had supplemented her understanding of surgery through simulations. Still, when Dr. Harding handed her the scalpel and said, “Your turn,” Lucy’s hands trembled.

“I—I don’t think I’m ready.”

“You won’t ever feel ready. Just start.”

The incision was hesitant, her suturing slow and clumsy. But she did it. It didn't matter that Dr. Harding did everything in-between. She performed as necessary after seeing only one procedure.

Afterward, in the break room, she sat staring at her hands.

Dr. Harding leaned against the counter. "You think I actually meant SODOTO literally?"

Lucy looked up, confused.

"See one, do one, teach one—people think it means you watch once, then you're on your own. That's nonsense." He crossed his arms. "You've seen dozens of appendectomies, read about hundreds, and practiced on cadavers and simulations. You're doing them now, under supervision. And someday, when you teach, you'll still be learning. That's what it really means."

Lucy absorbed his words. It wasn't about perfection. It was about progress.

Her six-week rotation flew by. She completed her time under Dr. Harding's watchful eye, gaining confidence but still yearning for more. When the opportunity arose in her fourth year for an elective in general surgery, she signed up immediately, requesting Dr. Harding's team.

When she returned, the OR felt familiar rather than daunting.

"Back for more, Knapp?" Dr. Harding asked, a glint of approval in his eyes.

This time, she wasn't the nervous student escaping to the back of the room. She was assisting, handling instruments with surer hands. Watching from the periphery was a third-year medical student—wide-eyed, anxious, reminding Lucy so much of herself just a year ago.

After a routine cholecystectomy, Dr. Harding turned to Lucy. "Why don't you walk our new student through what we just did?"

Lucy hesitated, then exhaled. "Sure," she said. Turning to the student, she began explaining step by step. She wasn't just watching anymore. She wasn't just doing it.

She was teaching.

Years later, an accomplished surgeon herself, Dr. Lucy Knapp would always introduce herself to anxious patients and family members the same way: “I’m Dr. Knapp. The ‘K’ is silent—but not like me.”

And she had Dr. Harding to thank for that.

43. Work, Love, and Play

A psychiatrist supplies the necessary ingredients for a rewarding medical marriage.

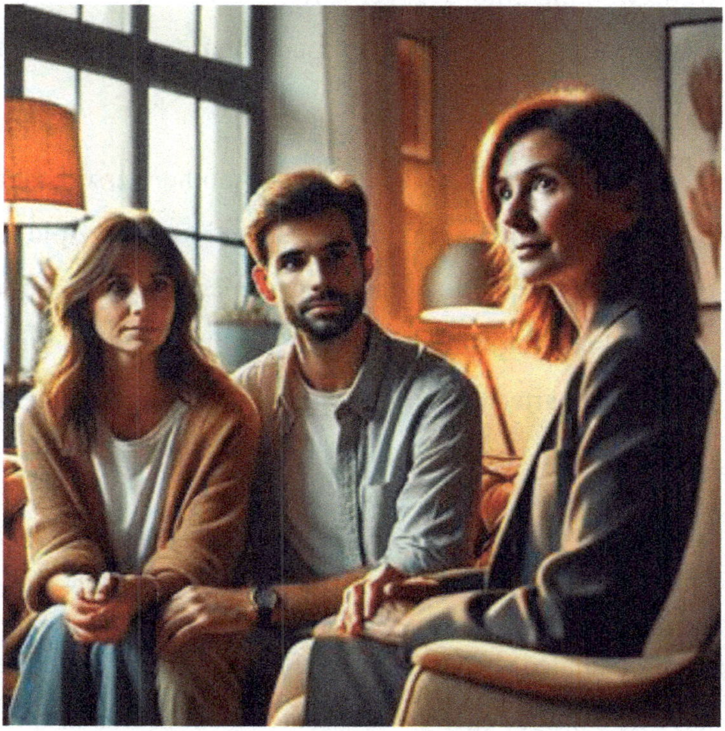

Dr. Loretta Stern glanced at the clock on the car's dashboard as she pulled into the parking lot. 6:58 p.m. Two minutes until their first couples' therapy session.

Dr. Robbie Spellman pouted next to her, massaging his temples. "I can't believe we're doing this."

"Neither can I," Loretta admitted.

They had managed to find a last-minute babysitter for their one-year-old son, Max, so at least they didn't have to juggle childcare on top of everything else tonight. Still, walking into a psychiatrist's office felt foreign, even for two physicians who spent their days immersed in patient care.

Dr. Layla Blumenthal was a working mother herself. Her office was warm and inviting, designed to put people at ease. She possessed an easy confidence, greeting them with a knowing smile. Her auburn hair, tinged with silver, was parted on the side, and she exuded the kind of calm that made people want to talk.

She motioned for them to sit. "So," she began, her voice warm and calm. "Tell me why you're here."

Loretta inhaled sharply. "Honestly? We're drowning. We have no time for each other. Medical school was insane, residency almost broke us, and now it feels like we're living in a pressure cooker. Everything is work—at the hospital, at home, everywhere. It's all just logistics, task lists, and schedules. I'd rather be a musician living my life on the road—too busy to make plans."

Robbie let out a humorless chuckle. "Logistics? Try survival." He rubbed a hand down his face. "I work 60-hour weeks, come home to a baby who doesn't sleep, and a wife who's—" He hesitated.

"A wife who's what?" Loretta pressed, narrowing her eyes.

"A wife who's just as exhausted as I am," he muttered. "We don't have time for anything. No time to talk, no time to sleep, no time to—"

"Be married?" Dr. Blumenthal finished.

He nodded, exhaling.

Loretta looked down at her lap. "We thought things would get better after residency. That once we had jobs, a home, a routine, things would chill."

"But they didn't," Dr. Blumenthal observed.

Robbie smirked, shaking his head. "Nope. If anything, they got worse."

Dr. Blumenthal leaned forward slightly. "You're both high-achieving, driven people. That's what got you through med school, through residency, through everything that's been thrown at you so far. But let me ask you this—when was the last time you had fun together?"

Loretta blinked. "Fun?"

"Yes," Dr. Blumenthal said. "Not just sitting on the couch exhausted after a long day, not tag-teaming childcare or errands. Actual fun. Laughing, enjoying each other's company, doing something just because it felt good."

They were eerily silent. Finally, Lorette broke the ice.

"I don't even know. Our wedding? Our honeymoon?"

"That was almost five years ago," Dr. Blumenthal pointed out gently.

Robbie shifted uncomfortably.

She continued, "You know, Freud once said that the key to psychological well-being is finding balance between work and love. Someone later added a third ingredient—play. Work, love, and play. The three things human beings need to be fulfilled and well-adjusted. And the more complex the mind, the more need for fun."

Robbie frowned. “Well, we’ve got the work part covered. And love… I mean, we love each other; we love our son.”

“But no fun,” Dr. Blumenthal said simply.

Robbie exhaled. “Who has time to play?”

Loretta shook her head. “I don’t even know what we’d do for fun anymore.”

Dr. Blumenthal smiled knowingly. “Exactly. You’ve spent so long building a life together that you forgot to live in it.”

Loretta swallowed hard, staring at the floor.

Robbie rubbed his jaw, looking over at her. “So, what, we just go on a date night and magically fix everything?”

Dr. Blumenthal chuckled. “I wouldn’t go that far. But I would suggest finding moments—small ones, even—to inject a little levity back into your relationship. Not everything has to be so serious. Some days, I just lean into the chaos, write a lengthy to-do list that I promptly lose somewhere in my house, and try to laugh at the many indignities of aging.”

Loretta felt a small, unexpected chuckle rise in her throat.

Robbie smirked. “So, your solution is…laughter?”

“No,” Dr. Blumenthal said. “But it helps.” She studied them both before continuing. “You’ve spent so long just trying to survive. I want to help you reconnect—not just as co-parents or co-homeowners, but as Loretta and Robbie, the people who chose each other.”

***

The room fell silent.

Dr. Blumenthal checked the time. “That’s all for tonight.”

Loretta’s eyes widened. Already?

Robbie, too, was unaware how fast the time had passed. “That’s it? What’s our homework?”

Dr. Blumenthal smiled. “No homework. Just…pay attention. To yourselves, to each other. And maybe, if the moment presents itself, find some time to play or something to laugh about.”

As they walked to the car, Loretta reached for the door handle, then hesitated. She glanced at Robbie.

He shook his head. "I still don't know if this is going to help."

Loretta clicked on her seatbelt. "Well, it's more than we were doing before."

Robbie grunted in reluctant agreement.

Then, after a pause, he smirked. "You know, I can't believe she admitted to losing her to-do lists. I mean—"

They both looked at each other and smiled. Loretta chuckled, shaking her head. "Maybe laughter really is the answer."

Robbie reached for her hand, giving it a small squeeze.

Perhaps they weren't completely lost yet.

44. A Dose of Reality

One doctor provides another a glimpse into the commercial world of pharmaceutical marketing.

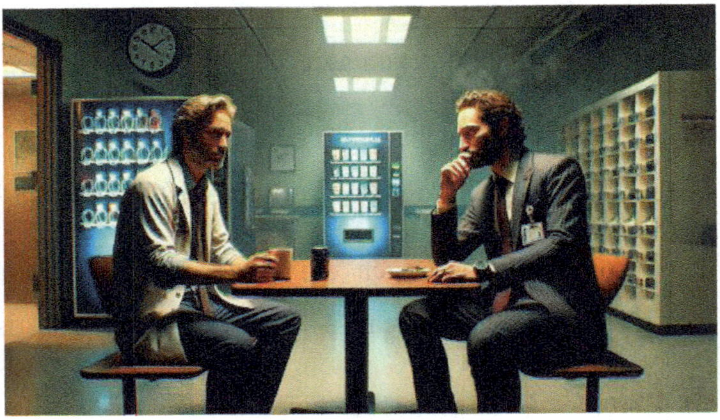

Dr. Holden Grudge sat in the dimly lit break room of Prophet Medical Center, his coffee turning cold as he stared into space. He had just finished seeing his last patient of the day—another patient filled with unrealistic expectations fueled by drug commercials.

Dr. Ben E. Fitts, a neatly dressed pharmaceutical liaison with a winning smile, strode in, adjusting his designer tie. “Dr. Grudge,” he said cheerfully. “Always a pleasure. How’s your day treating you?"

Grudge let out a sigh. “I’m beside myself, Fitts.”

Fitts pulled up a chair, his polished leather shoes reflecting the overhead light. “If you’re feeling overwhelmed or stressed, it might be helpful to talk about what’s going on.”

Grudge shot him a look. “You want to help? You’re part of the problem. Can you explain these TV drug commercials? My patients don’t know what any of these diseases or drug classes are—just a jumble of letters: AFib, IBS-C, wet AMD, JAK inhibitors, GLP-1s, and SGLT-2s. It’s like alphabet soup, but with a terrible aftertaste.”

Fitts chuckled. “I understand the frustration. But the commercials are meant to educate consumers about available treatments.”

“Educate?” Grudge barked a laugh. “They baffle patients into thinking they need some miracle drug with a name that sounds like a rejected Star Wars character. Next thing you know, they’re in my office demanding it.”

Fitts leaned forward, his hands steepled. “Patients deserve to know their options. And let’s be honest, they’re going to look up symptoms and drugs online anyway. Wouldn't you rather they get information from a regulated source?"

Grudge shook his head. "You mean the commercials where a lady twirls in a sunlit meadow while a soothing voice warns she might experience nausea, dizziness, liver failure, or sudden death?"

Fitts smiled. "Balance, Dr. Grudge. The FDA requires fair presentation of risks and benefits."

"Fair?" Grudge scoffed. "The benefits are in bold print. The risks are rattled off like an auctioneer selling used cars." He leaned in. "The real problem is that my patients come in convinced these drugs will work miracles. And half the time, they're not even appropriate candidates."

Fitts nodded sympathetically. "That's why patient education is key. We encourage dialogue between doctors and patients."

Grudge threw up his hands. "Great. And when I finally convince them they don't need the drug, they realize they can't afford it anyway. Have you seen the prices of those biologics?"

Fitts cleared his throat. "I won't deny some specialty drugs are expensive. But we offer patient assistance programs, copay cards—"

Grudge cut him off. "Yeah, if you're two standard deviations below the poverty level. And insurance? Ha! They won't cover these drugs unless my patients have 'failed' cheaper, less effective alternatives first. You know what failing means, Fitts? It means suffering. It means coming back sicker, desperate, and with fewer options left."

Fitts sighed. "The system isn't perfect, but—"

"But?" Grudge snapped. "But what? You'll keep selling the dream while I deal with the reality? Let me ask you something."

"Anything, sure."

"Where is the medical muscle in your company? You're a doctor, after all. Why don't you push back against those marketing teams? Hell, they don't care about patients. All they want to do is rake in the dollars for the company and be recognized as a 'rising star.'"

Fitts let out a long sigh. "I tried pushing back, Grudge. Look where it got me. Demoted to a medical liaison.

Traveling most of the time, away from my family, acting like a huckster dealing with—"

"I know," Grudge said softly. "Schmucks like me."

"Well—"

"It's okay, Fitts. I'm not offended. Hell, I've even thought about working for pharma myself. Tell me, what happened to get you demoted?"

Fitts was surprised at the question, but he seemed genuinely happy to answer it. "First, I confronted a VP. I told her she was making a mistake by denying funding for a well-thought-out research proposal submitted by a KOL."

"KOL?" Grudge? asked, perplexed by the term.

"Key Opinion Leader," Fitts remarked, spelling it out. "Someone like you. A respected and influential doctor"—

"Hold on," Grudge barked. "No need to schmooze me to prescribe more of your company's drugs."

"No, really. It's a term we use with genuine intent to recognize your expertise and contributions to patient care and medical research. Your insights and endorsements can be highly valuable for companies looking to introduce new medical products or therapies to the market."

"Hmm...but that still doesn't answer my question about your demotion."

"Well," Fitts continued, "the VP called my manager and demanded I be fired for confronting her."

"Holy shit! Did she have the authority to do that?"

"Not really. And besides, my boss went to bat for me. But he told me to cool my jets with her. And you know what? We got along swimmingly from then on."

"So, why did they knock you down a rung?" Grudge persisted.

"I acted like a policeman."

"You...what!"

"I acted like a policeman—and I pissed everyone off. I was appointed to our promotional review committee, the one that reviews all drug advertising before it's released, the very drugs you see advertised on TV and in medical journals and doctors' waiting rooms."

"That sounds interesting," Grudge responded.

"I loved it, actually. The only problem was, I found too much wrong with the advertising—half-baked truths and funny numbers. You know: 'Lies, damn lies, and statistics'."

Grudge was familiar with that term from his biostatistics course in med school. "Lies, damn lies, and statistics," his professor proclaimed, a phrase of uncertain origin but nonetheless suggesting that numbers can be manipulated to support various arguments or viewpoints.

"I see," Grudge affirmed. "So that was your downfall?"

Fitts seemed determined to bring the conversation to an end. "The truth is, the company decided to replace me with a pharmacist. They said it was cheaper, that a pharmacist's eyes could substitute for those of a doctor. But we both know that's not true. Pharmacists are professional, alright, but they don't have the touch and feel for patient care like us, the nuanced understanding of what it's like to practice medicine… So here I am."

Grudge leaned back. He was incredulous at what he had just heard. Fitts spoke the truth like a real insider, a whistleblower. The two men seemed to bond over similar experiences fighting the establishment.

“I get it,” Grudge said. “The worst part for me is how I’m steamrolled by insurance companies, and I don’t even have the time to fight them. I’m drowning in paperwork while some AI algorithm denies my appeals. What kind of healthcare system does that"?

Fitts hesitated. “A complicated one,” he admitted. “Look, I don’t make the rules. But I do believe in innovation. AI contributes to drug R&D, and the drugs we develop do change lives.”

Grudge exhaled, staring at his empty coffee cup. “Yeah, no doubt, and those commercials come with catchy music that makes it sound like taking them is a cakewalk into wellness.”

Fitts chuckled. “Marketing, my friend.”

Grudge smirked. “You got a song for me, Fitts? Something upbeat to drown out this mess? Because right now, all I’m thinking about is James Taylor: ‘I’m a steamroller, baby. I'm ‘bout to roll all over you’.”

Fitts laughed and pulled out his phone. He began scrolling. “How about ‘Don’t Stop Believin’?”

Grudge shook his head, chuckling despite himself. “Fitting. The anthem for patients who think a pill will fix everything.”

Fitts smiled. “Or for doctors still holding out hope.”

Grudge sighed, then stood up, stretching. “If I ever find that hope, Fitts, I’ll let you know.”

As he walked out, Fitts called after him, “I’ll be waiting, Dr. Grudge.”

Grudge waved a hand without looking back. “Yeah, yeah. Don’t hold your breath.”

And with that, he disappeared down the hall, leaving Fitts alone with the quiet drumming of the vending machine and the irony of their conversation lingering in the air, both of them defeated by the system.

Later that night, as Grudge sank into his sofa with iTunes in hand, he scrolled past Journey’s “Don’t Stop Believin’” without a second thought. Instead, he let Bob Marley’s voice fill the room. “Three Little Birds” played softly, Grudge whispering the lyrics out loud—‘Don’t worry about a thing. ‘Cause every little thing gonna be alright’—letting the message wash over him like a prescription he wasn’t sure would work.

45. Signs, Signs, Every where a Sign

A physician is made aware that compassion, communication, and common sense belong in a conversation—not on a wall.

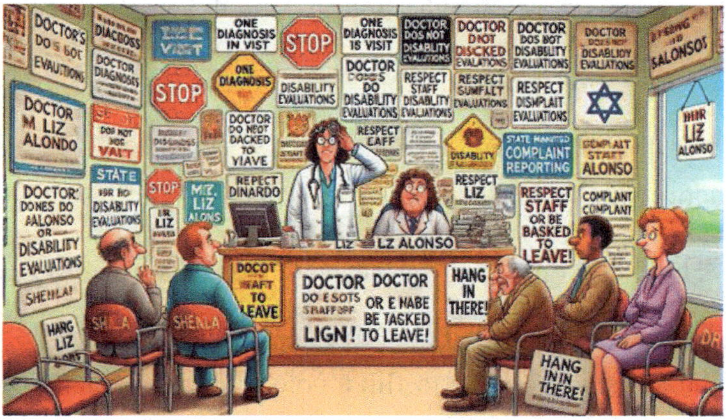

Dr. Liz Alonso moaned as she walked through a crowded waiting room, juggling her coffee, stethoscope, and a tablet that had mysteriously disappeared by the time she got to her office. The receptionist, Sheila, greeted her with a wide grin.

"Brace yourself, Doc," Sheila said, tilting her head toward Room 3. "Mr. DiNardo saw The Sign."

Liz groaned. The sign had been up for two weeks, and it had already caused more outrage than a hospital cafeteria running out of coffee.

She took a deep breath, pushed open the exam room door, and stepped into the battlefield.

“Ah, Dr. Alonso,” Mr. DiNardo said, arms crossed. “Do you happen to know what’s written on the window of the receptionist’s office?”

Liz nodded slowly. “I assume you mean the sign about addressing one primary diagnosis per visit?”

“That’s the one! Do you hear yourself? One diagnosis per visit! How does that even work? If I have a cough and a rash, do I have to flip a coin to decide which one you’ll acknowledge today?”

Liz pinched the bridge of her nose. “Mr. DiNardo—”

“No, no, let’s really think this through,” he interrupted, eyes gleaming with the kind of passion normally reserved for sports debates. “Is shortness of breath and chest pain one problem or two? What if I trip down the stairs and break my wrist and my ankle? Will I simply wrap one like a burrito and leave the other hanging until next week?

Sheila knocked on the door and poked her head in, smiling at Mr. DiNardo. "Just a heads up, Doc. Mrs. Donnelly read the 'Doctor does not do disability evaluations' sign and is currently composing a very detailed online review."

Liz exhaled. "Great."

"Yeah, and a guy in the waiting room said he's been reading walls in clinics for 15 years and enough is enough." Sheila lowered her voice. "He also suggested we replace all signs with motivational cat posters."

Mr. DiNardo waved a hand. "See? People are fed up! Signs, signs, everywhere a sign. It's all messages like 'Don't ask too many questions,' 'Don't expect too much,' and 'Whatever you do, do not complain.'"

Liz sighed. "It's not meant to be like that. The sign is just"… She hesitated.

"A symptom of a larger problem?" he offered.

"For sure," she admitted. "Volume drives revenue. More patients, more visits. It's not personal—it's corporate."

He wagged a finger. "There's the problem! Medicine is becoming transactional. You know what happens when you try to separate symptoms into neat little boxes? Misdiagnoses, delays, frustration. You can't force medicine into a one-size-fits-all model."

Liz groaned. "I know. But I don't make the rules."

"So why not push back?" Mr. DiNardo leaned forward. "Here's my idea: instead of these cold, passive-aggressive signs, how about something useful? Maybe a friendly infographic? A pamphlet? Heck, I'd take a 'Choose Your Own Adventure' book at this point."

Liz chuckled. "I do like the idea of replacing them with cat posters."

Sheila reappeared. "Speaking of which, someone just added a sticky note under the 'One Diagnosis Per Visit' sign that says, 'How about one good diagnosis per visit?' And they underlined good."

Liz buried her face in her hands. "I give up."

Mr. DiNardo grinned. "See, Doc? Patients want communication, not bureaucracy. We don't need signage telling us to behave or be silent. We need doctors who listen."

Liz nodded slowly. "You make a fair point." She turned to Sheila. "Okay, take down The Sign. Let's replace it with something… I don't know, human."

Sheila raised an eyebrow. "Like what?"

Liz thought for a moment, then smirked. *"How about: 'Your health is complicated, and we get it. We'll do our best today—if we need more time, we'll figure it out together.'"*

Mr. DiNardo beamed. "Now that's a sign I'd actually read."

Then he frowned. "Wait a second… What about all the other signs? The ones about reporting doctors? The warnings about respecting staff? The laundry list of patient responsibilities and rights?"

Liz rubbed her temples. "Some of those are state-mandated, Mr. DiNardo. Many states require doctors to post signage directing patients to complaint boards or licensing agencies. If we don't, we can actually get fined."

Mr. DiNardo threw up his hands. "So, the state forces you to clutter up the walls with bureaucratic nonsense?"

Liz shrugged. "Pretty much."

He stood up and grabbed his coat. "Well, I'll tell you one thing, Doc. I am going to file a complaint."

Liz blinked. "A complaint about what?"

Mr. DiNardo grinned. "About the requirement for all these ridiculous signs! Maybe they need a sign reminding them that patients are people, not paperwork."

Liz watched him march out of the office, shaking her head with a chuckle.

She turned to Sheila. "Think we can get away with replacing everything with a single poster that just says, 'Welcome. We're here to help. Let's *talk'*.

Sheila smirked. "Only if it has a cat on it."

Liz sighed. "Fine. But I'm picking the cat."

46. My Stressed-Out (Wonderful) Life

A doctor finds refuge in family, faith, and Friday nights.

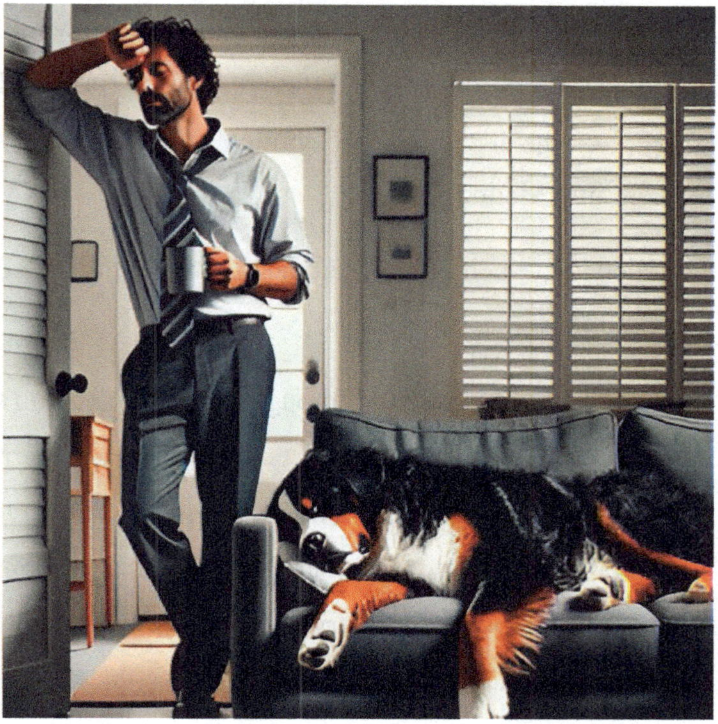

Dr. Noam Himmelstein stood in the doorway of his living room, coffee in one hand, tie hanging loosely from his unbuttoned collar. His shoulders sagged under the invisible weight of the day ahead. On the dark gray sofa, his Bernese Mountain Dog, Baxter, was sprawled in a perfect picture of bliss—limbs akimbo, head buried in a pillow, one ear flopped over as if gravity had lost interest.

Noam let out a dry chuckle. "Must be nice, huh?"

Baxter didn't so much as flick an ear in acknowledgment.

"If I wrote a book about my life, you know what it would be called? My Stressed-Out Life." Noam took a sip of coffee, staring at the dog. "Subtitle: A Nephrologist's Descent into Madness."

The silence, broken only by Baxter's soft snoring, filled the room like an accusation.

Noam sighed and ran a hand through his hair. "You don't have to deal with pre-rounds at 6:30 AM. Or an intern who thinks 'AKI' stands for 'Always Keep Ignoring.' Or a hospital administrator who sends urgent emails about reducing costs while I'm trying to keep someone's kidneys from shutting down."

Still nothing from Baxter.

"I bet you don't even dream about work. You probably dream about chasing rabbits or rolling in dirt. Meanwhile, I wake up in a cold sweat because I forgot to check someone's potassium level."

Noam’s phone buzzed in his pocket. He already knew it wasn’t good news. He glanced at the screen.

5:47 AM—Dr. Warner (Night Float)

Hey, sorry to bug you. 64-year-old M in MICU, post-contrast, Cr jumped from 1.1 to 3.4. Attending wants your take.

Noam exhaled through his nose. His temples throbbed. It was too early for this. Did they really need his opinion about contrast-induced nephropathy, a pretty common occurrence in hospitalized patients, usually reversible with proper supportive care?

“Of course,” he muttered. “Because nothing says good morning like a textbook case of iatrogenic kidney injury.” He typed back a quick response.

On my way.

Noam turned back to Baxter, who was still deeply committed to his long night's sleep.

“You know, buddy,” he murmured, “maybe in my next life, I’ll come back as you. No EMRs. No burnout. No PTSD in my residency.”

His voice softened. “Just...peace.”

Baxter twitched a paw in his sleep, as if to agree.

Noam sighed and tightened his tie. "Alright. Time to go be a doctor."

He grabbed his bag, ran a hand over Baxter's fur—soft, warm, real—and walked out the door.

***

Dr. Noam Himmelstein pulled into the driveway just as the last traces of daylight melted into a deep indigo sky. He turned off the car and sat for a moment, inhaling the stillness. For once, he was home at a decent hour, on a Friday night no less. Shabbat.

Inside, the house was alive with warmth. The scent of freshly baked challah and simmering brisket wrapped around him like an embrace. Laughter tumbled from the dining room, where the glow of candles flickered against the walls.

"Noam! Just in time!" called his wife, Miriam, from the kitchen. She peeked around the corner, her apron dusted with flour, and gave him the kind of smile that could make the whole week's stress seem like an afterthought.

From the dining room, their 12-year-old son, Jonah, looked up from his Bar Mitzvah invitation list. "Abba, you have to help! Mom thinks 300 guests is "a little much'." He said this with dramatic air quotes.

"A little much?" Miriam appeared at Noam's side, raising an eyebrow. "Noam, do we even know 300 people?"

"I'm a doctor, honey. You know how many kidneys I've saved? That's got to count for something." He shrugged off his coat and gave her a quick kiss. "Besides, if it were up to your mother, we'd be having an intimate gathering of, what, fifty people?"

Miriam smirked. "Seventy-five."

"That's a minyan and a half," their 10-year-old daughter, Talia, quipped as she set the table. "I think we should invite 500, just to be safe."

Jonah gasped. "Talia, you are my favorite sibling."

"I'm your only sibling."

"Exactly."

Laughter bubbled around the room as they took their seats. Noam, still in his work clothes, slid into his chair at the head of the table, feeling the tension of the week melt away. He recited Kiddush, savoring the rich sweetness of the wine, the way it anchored him to tradition, to home.

As Miriam tore the challah and passed it around, Jonah turned to Noam. "Abba, are you going to be stressed next week too?"

"Probably," Noam admitted, taking a bite of the warm bread. "But that's what this is for." He gestured around the table. "This…resets me."

Talia tilted her head. "Like a reboot?"

"You could say."

Miriam nudged him gently. "Then maybe next Friday, you'll get home early before I spend half an hour yelling at the kids to set the table?"

"Hey!" both kids protested in unison.

Noam chuckled. "No promises. But I'll try."

The night stretched on in a blur of good food and easy conversation, the kind that only happens when time slows and the world outside doesn't matter. They debated centerpiece colors for the Bar Mitzvah, whether they *really* needed a DJ *and* a live band (Jonah insisted they did), and how much kugel was too much kugel (the consensus: there was no such thing).

Eventually, one by one, the family retired for the night.

Except Baxter.

The big Bernese Mountain Dog lay stretched out near the dining table, staring expectantly at Noam, his eyebrows lifting in a way that said, *You forgot something, human.*

Noam closed his eyes, remembering. “Oh no.”

Baxter thumped his tail.

“The kids forgot to give you challah, didn’t they?”

A single, dramatic sigh from Baxter confirmed it.

Noam chuckled, breaking off a small piece from the remaining loaf. “Here you go, buddy. Can’t have you missing out on Shabbat.”

Baxter took it gently, chewing with exaggerated satisfaction. Then, instead of trotting off, he nudged Noam’s knee, his massive head and body leaning into his leg the way only a Berner can.

Noam ran a hand over Baxter’s thick fur, feeling his warmth, his presence, and his unwavering love. “Fine, you win. Extra love it is." He rubbed behind Baxter's ears, his fingers sinking into soft fur as Baxter let out a deep, contented sigh.

For a long moment, Noam just sat there, his hand resting on his dog, the house quiet, the week's stress nothing more than a distant memory.

"Alright," he murmured finally, giving Baxter one last scratch. "Go be a dog."

Baxter gave him one last, satisfied lean before padding off toward his bed.

And Noam, buoyed by the love of his family, the warmth of tradition, and the unshakable presence of his loyal dog, finally did the same.

If he ever decided to write that book, he thought, slipping into bed beside his already sleeping beautiful Miriam, he would change the title to My Stressed-Out Wonderful Life.

Then he turned the light out.

47. Stand Up for Science

A doctor fights broken promises with unbroken purpose.

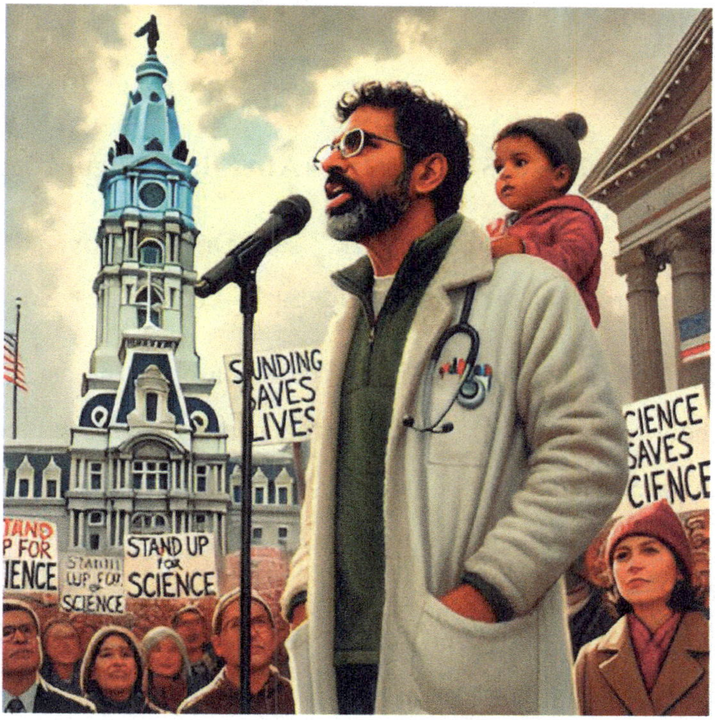

March 7, 2025

The crowd outside City Hall swelled like a rising tide. Homemade signs bobbed in the sea of people: *"In Science We Trust," "Data Over Dogma,"* and "Funding Saves Lives." Chants rang out in waves. Somewhere near the edge of the speaker's platform, Dr. Renga Choudhary stood, unmoving.

His original intention was not to speak.

But sometimes the world rearranges your silence into a scream.

***

January 25, 2025 — Five Days After the Inauguration

"Renga, the scan came back," said Dr. Ames over the speakerphone. "It's pancreatic. Early—but aggressive."

Across the kitchen, Shreya's eyes searched his as she held their daughter, Meena, on her lap. Renga steadied himself against the counter.

"What are our options?"

"There's a new trial—T3-CAR therapy. Targets the KRAS mutation. The university is enrolling".

"Then let's do it," Renga said without hesitation.

But five days later, the headlines struck first:

NIH Cuts 117 Active Trials as New Administration Orders Immediate Budget Freeze.

And an email followed.

Dear Dr. Choudhary, Due to a sudden funding suspension, the T3-CAR trial has been placed on indefinite hold. We deeply regret the impact this may have on your family.

Renga stared at the screen, jaw clenched. His silence no longer felt noble. It felt complicit.

***

February 1, 2025

At the kitchen table, Shreya's infusion pump ticked softly. Meena colored beside her, the crayons moving in rhythmic, distracted circles.

"I didn't come to this country to watch it betray itself," Renga murmured.

Shreya met his eyes. "You always believed in quiet service."

He nodded. "But quiet's not working anymore."

***

February 18, 2025

At his modest office, Renga's day began like any other—chart reviews, a Pap smear, and a diabetic foot exam. But at 2:04 PM, he got a text from his niece:

ICE van seen on 7th Street near Uncle Ramesh's place. Warn him.

His brother-in-law, Ramesh, was a legal resident. An engineer. His only misstep: signing a petition demanding the restoration of NIH grants halted in the executive orders of late January.

Renga sat down hard in the break room. *They were coming for people like him. Like Shreya. Like his entire family tree.*

***

March 1, 2025

The flyer arrived via email: **"STAND UP FOR SCIENCE—March 7 Rally at City Hall."**

He almost deleted it.

Instead, he opened a reply window.

I am Dr. Renga Choudhary. I trained in India and have practiced medicine here for 20 years. I would like to speak—not just as a doctor, but as a husband and an immigrant. Science saved my patients...

He hesitated. The next words lodged in his throat.

It could save my wife…or…it could have saved my wife. Renga was unsure what tense to use.

***

March 7, 2025 — Rally Day

"Next up," the emcee called into the microphone, "is someone whose story reminds us all what's at stake. Please welcome Dr. Renga Choudhary."

As Renga stepped to the mic, the wind tugged at his coat. His voice came slow but clear.

"I came to this country with two suitcases and a stethoscope. I believed in its promise—that if you worked hard and served others, you'd be protected."

He paused, scanning the sea of faces.

"My wife, Shreya, was diagnosed with pancreatic cancer two weeks after the new administration took office. The therapy with the highest potential to save her—a trial funded by your tax dollars—was abruptly frozen by executive order. Not because it failed science. Because it failed politics."

Ripples of dismay moved through the crowd.

"I've spent decades treating people from every walk of life. And I can tell you: science doesn't care about borders. Cancer doesn't care about immigration status. And neither should our funding priorities."

He drew in a breath.

"My brother-in-law now fears deportation—not for breaking laws, but for signing a petition. My daughter, five years old, now asks if Mommy will die because someone in Washington doesn't like her or believe in science."

His voice cracked.

"I believed in quiet service. I stayed out of politics. But when science is under siege, silence is not neutrality—it's surrender."

He looked up.

"I will not stand idly by while research is gutted, while immigrants are silenced, while my wife suffers for a therapy that exists—but has been buried."

He lifted a hand, trembling but resolute.

"Shreya once told me that quiet doesn't save lives. Speaking does. Funding does. Science does."

The crowd erupted.

***

Later That Evening

Meena was curled on the couch, a crayon sign still clutched in her fingers: *"Science Saved My Amma."*

Shreya smiled weakly from her recliner, fatigue dimming her eyes but not her fire. "You did well today."

Renga sank beside her, forehead to hers. "I should've done it sooner."

She whispered, "You did it now. That's what counts."

***

Epilogue — Weeks After the Rally

The T3-CAR trial was resurrected by an emergency grant from a private foundation inspired by the March 7 protests. Shreya began treatment soon thereafter.

Renga kept practicing—but now he also spoke. On campuses. In D.C. In the press.

He had once been the quiet doctor with the gentle eyes. Now, he was the voice that stood up for science—and never sat down again.

48. Press 4 for Drama.

A doctor and pharmacist interact in a most unpleasant way.

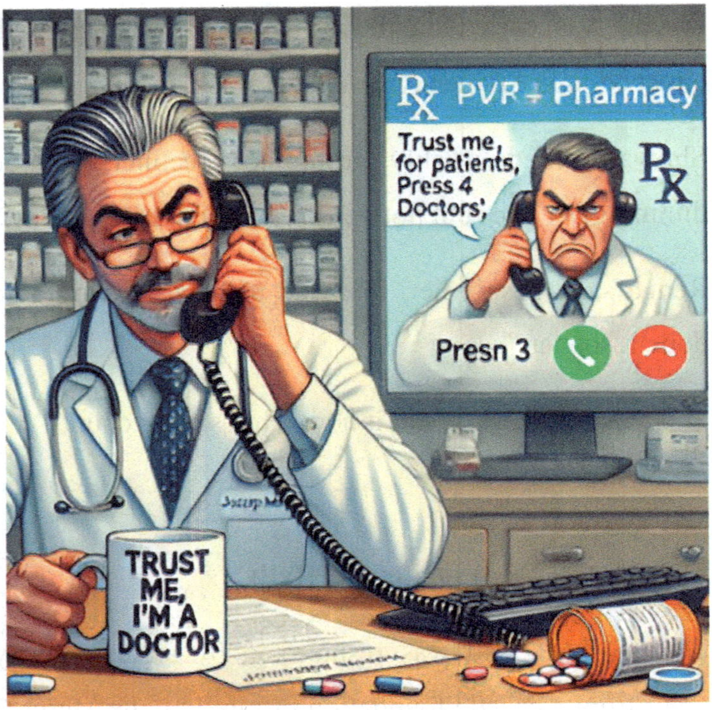

Dr. Joseph Mason had a theory about pharmacy IVR systems.

"They're not built for efficiency," he once told his medical assistant. "They're built to test your blood pressure medication."

One Saturday morning, sitting in his home office with a cup of coffee and a to-do list, already muttering threats, he attempted to refill his lorazepam prescription. Low-dose, 0.5 mg tablets, prescribed by his own primary care physician for occasional insomnia. Routine. Nothing suspicious.

He called Happy Well Pharmacy.

"Thank you for calling Happy Well Pharmacy! For store hours, press 1. To speak to a pharmacist, press 2. For prescription refills, press 3. If you are a doctor or representing a doctor's office, press 4..."

He pressed 3.

The system prompted him to enter the prescription number. He typed it in slowly, precisely.

"Four... five... nine... eight..."

"Thank you. Please hold while we access your information—"

Click.

The line went dead.

Joseph sighed. "Shocking."

He redialed. Same outcome.

Next time he pressed 4. The doctor's line.

A click. Then a voice. Gruff. Irritated.

"Doctors line. This is Dale."

"Hi Dale, this is Joseph Mason. I'm calling about a renewal —"

"You're calling the doctor's hotline."

Joseph blinked. "Yes. I am a doctor."

A pause. Dale didn't laugh. Instead, he continued, "This line isn't for routine stuff. It's for urgent care coordination, clinical exceptions, and real-time consultation. Not patient refills."

"I tried the refill line. It crashed. Twice. This is my only shot at human contact."

Dale sounded unconvinced. "What are you trying to fill?"

"Lorazepam."

Another pause.

"Fine. I see it," Dale said. "I'll process it now. But next time, use the patient line. Like everyone else."

"If the system stops booting me like a suspicious login, I will."

Click.

Two weeks later, an envelope arrived bearing the seal of the State Medical Licensing Board.

Joseph opened it and stared.

Subject: Notice of Investigation—Allegation of Self-Prescribing Controlled Substances

"You're kidding me," he muttered.

***

The Medical Board office was sterile and quiet. Joseph sat upright, professionally dressed but inwardly fuming. He had brought an empty bottle bearing the name of his PCP as the prescriber.

A door opened.

"Dr. Mason?" asked the assistant.

He followed her to a small conference room where a man in a charcoal suit stood.

"Michael Abrams. Investigator. Thanks for coming."

They shook hands.

"We received a complaint alleging potential self-prescription of lorazepam," Abrams said.

"Prescribed by Dr. Alexis Tran. My primary care physician. I'm the patient, not the prescriber."

Abrams nodded. "We've verified the prescription source. No red flags. No overuse. Sorry to have troubled you, but we needed to inform you in person."

"Do I get to know who reported it?"

"The source must remain anonymous. But we know."

***

One week later, the board convened again. This time, the subject of review was pharmacist Dale Strickland.

Dr. Yoon, the board chair, addressed the room.

"We have concerns about your recent complaint against Dr. Joseph Mason."

Dale straightened in his seat. "Pharmacists are allowed to refuse prescriptions at their discretion or report anything suspicious."

"Suspicious based on what?" asked a board member. "It was a low-dose benzodiazepine prescribed by another physician. Your only interaction was a phone call."

Dale stiffened. “He used the doctor’s line to refill lorazepam. It didn’t sit right with me.”

“So, your concern was the phone extension he pressed?”

Another member added, “That’s not clinical judgment. That’s personal retaliation.”

Dr. Yoon leaned forward. “We remind all licensees: discretion must be exercised responsibly. Not as cover for grievance.”

***

The board closed its investigation. Two letters went out.

Joseph’s read:

Your case has been closed. No further action is required. Thank you for your cooperation.

Dale’s read:

Following review, the board issues a formal reprimand for misuse of the complaint process. You are required to complete a CE course on ethics and discretionary reporting within 90 days.

At the bottom:

Discretion is the servant of judgment—not the mask of bias.

***

Weeks later, Joseph dropped by HappyWell Pharmacy for a flu shot. Dale was behind the counter.

Their eyes met. Silence.

“They’ll call you when they’re ready,” Dale said flatly.

Joseph nodded politely. “Appreciate it.”

The IVR sign above the counter had been updated:

Doctors with prescription questions: Press 4.

Refilling your own medication? Press 3 is preferred. But we won’t bite if you press 4.

Dr. Mason smiled.

49. The Edge of the Map

Some doctors wait for life to happen. Others chart their own course.

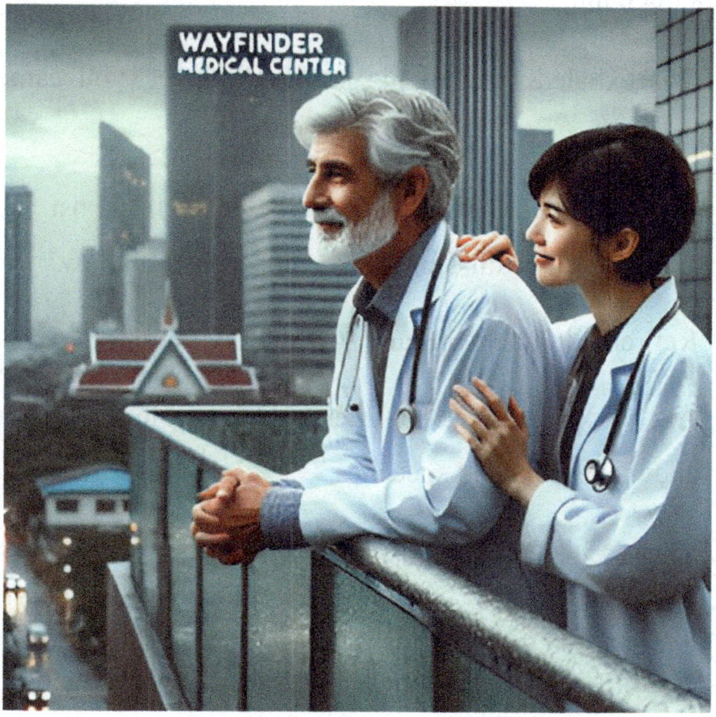

Dr. Elias Mercer stood on the rooftop of Wayfinder Medical Center, the city sprawled out before him like an unrolled map. The air was thick with the scent of approaching rain, but he didn't move. He just stood, hands clasped over the railing, staring out as though searching for something beyond the skyline.

Footsteps behind him. He didn't need to turn to know who it was.

"Should've known I'd find you up here," Dr. Olivia Cho said, stepping forward, her white coat billowing slightly in the wind.

Elias exhaled through his nose. "And yet, you came anyway."

Olivia smirked. "It's a gift." She leaned against the railing. "You're missing your own party, you know."

"Retirement luncheons aren't really my thing."

"Ah, yes. The great Dr. Mercer, too noble for finger sandwiches and bad speeches."

He gave her a sidelong glance. "You're enjoying this, aren't you?"

"A little." She nudged him with her elbow. "Come on. I thought you'd be the last person to go out like this—brooding on a rooftop instead of celebrating."

Elias didn't answer right away. He drummed his fingers against his knee, still watching the horizon. "You ever hear about those old maps? The ones where cartographers would mark the unknown with 'Here Be Dragons'?"

Olivia frowned. "What about them?"

"That's what this feels like. After today, the map runs out. No more schedule, no more cases, no more being needed at 3 a.m." His voice was quiet, distant. "I spent my whole life chasing something. But now? Now I don't even know what the chase is supposed to be."

Olivia looked at him. "So, you're telling me that after a career of tackling everything head-on, you're just…stopping?"

He gave a small, humorless chuckle. "Maybe. Maybe I've been running so long I don't know how to stop without falling flat on my face."

Olivia folded her arms. "You ever hear of Dr. Keltner?"

Elias glanced at her. "The endocrinologist?"

She nodded. "Retired three years ago. Had all these plans—travel, family, hobbies. You know what he does now?"

Elias raised a brow.

"He sits on his porch, drinking iced tea, watching the world go by. At first, he said he was enjoying the peace. But then something changed. He started talking about how he felt…smaller. Like his world was shrinking around him." Olivia turned toward him. "And you know what I think? I think people either meet life head-on, take hold of it, and make something of it—or they turn away from it, let it pass them by, and they start to wither."

Elias was silent.

"You, Elias Mercer, were never the type to wither."

He let the words sit between them, rolling them over in his mind. The wind picked up slightly, tugging at the edges of his coat.

Finally, he let out a breath. "I used to tell my residents something, you know."

Olivia raised an eyebrow.

"I'd tell them medicine's not about waiting for the right moment. It's about stepping up, doing the thing that needs doing before hesitation takes over."

She smirked. "And yet, here you are, hesitating."

Elias huffed out a laugh. "You're insufferable."

"And you love it—and I love you, my good friend," Olivia said, her voice softer now.

Elias turned to her fully, his eyes misty. He blinked a few times, then exhaled. "Well…that settles it, then. Can't have you thinking I'd let myself wither away."

Olivia smiled. "Darn right you can't."

He shook his head, a small chuckle escaping. "What do you think I should do?"

Olivia shrugged. "That's not my decision. But if it were me? I'd figure out what's left on the map. And if there's nothing there, I'd pick up a damn pen and draw more of it."

Elias considered that.

A drop of rain landed on his sleeve. Then another.

Olivia pushed off the railing. "Come inside. At least pretend to enjoy your party."

Elias looked out over the city one last time, then stood, rolling his shoulders back. "Yeah," he murmured, more to himself than to her. "Alright."

And as he followed her inside, he realized that perhaps his best work wasn't behind him.

Maybe there was still more map left to draw.

50. The Fifth Spring

Two frontline physicians rehash the COVID-19 pandemic and question the future.

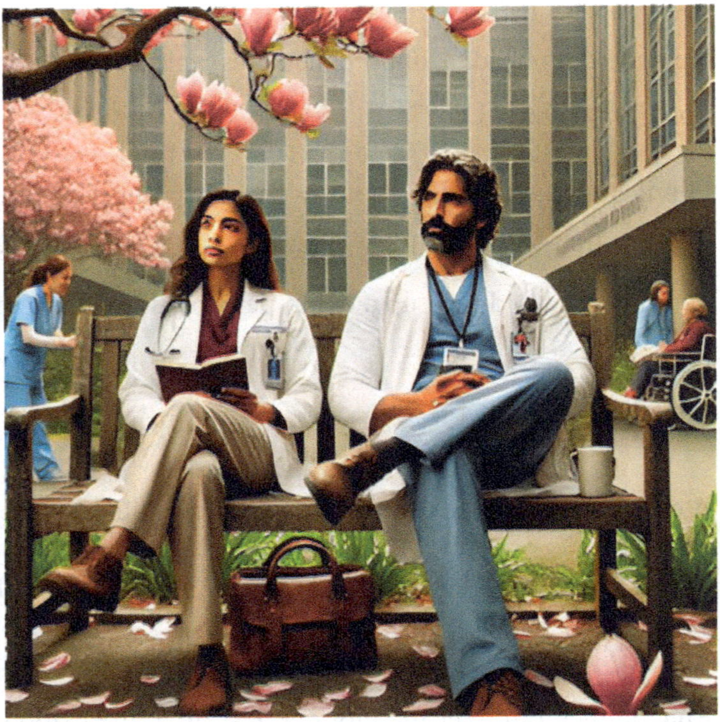

The magnolias were blooming early this spring, their pale pink petals fluttering down onto the worn brick pathway outside the hospital courtyard. Dr. Eva Cardenas wrapped her thin white coat tighter as she waited on a bench, the same one she used to eat lunch on during the worst months of 2020, six feet apart from everyone else. She'd brought coffee in a flask—two mugs—and a memory she wasn't sure she wanted to share.

Dr. Rajiv Menon arrived ten minutes late, still with the same brisk, clipped walk, but now a little slower, his salt-and-pepper beard fuller. He saw her and smiled, a little sadly.

"Five years," he said, sitting down. "They call this an anniversary? Five years since the lockdown? It feels like both yesterday and someone else's lifetime ago."

"Maybe both," Eva replied, pouring coffee into the mugs. "You take sugar?"

"I used to," Rajiv said. "Stopped during the pandemic. Figured if I had to choose a vice, it'd be sleep deprivation instead."

They clinked mugs anyway.

For a few moments, they just sat, watching the sun spill onto the courtyard stones. Across from them stood the new wing of the hospital—state-of-the-art, LEED-certified, and born out of federal COVID relief funds. The irony wasn't lost on either of them.

"You know," Eva began, "I thought I'd feel more…resolved today. Like the anniversary would be some kind of closure."

Rajiv nodded. "I don't think medicine really does closure."

She glanced sideways at him. "But we were there, Rajiv. Every day. We saw it. The exhaustion. The tears. The bodies. All of it. And now, it's like it never happened."

"They remember the toilet paper shortages," he said, voice dry. "The school closures. The TikToks."

"But not the nights we had to bag three bodies before lunch," she murmured.

Silence again.

"I still remember that week in April," Rajiv said, "when we had to double up patients on ventilators. I didn't think that was even possible until we did it. And you—God, Eva, I still think about you running that code while your mom was on a vent two floors down."

Eva stared into her mug. "And yet...they talk about how the lockdowns ruined everything. The economy, education. And sure, they did a number. But they saved lives too."

"Hard truth," Rajiv said, "is that most people only mourn what touches them directly. We lost one in 300 Americans. And still no National Day of Mourning. No memorial."

"No reckoning," Eva added. "No real investment in public health. Just...scapegoating. Defunding. Conspiracies."

"You know what breaks me sometimes?" Rajiv asked. "That we showed up. Every damn day. When we didn't have enough PPE. When we didn't have treatment. When we didn't even know if the virus stayed on surfaces or floated in the air. We still came. And now we're just tired, burned out, or gone."

"Or worse—mistrusted," Eva added bitterly. "Remember when the vaccines came out? We thought it was the beginning of the end. But it turned into a referendum on truth."

"We trained for disease, Eva. Not disinformation."

They sat there as spring sunlight warmed their backs and the wind rustled the new leaves.

"But we did learn things," Eva said suddenly. "We learned that nurses are the backbone of every hospital. That teamwork means trusting someone to hold your life in their hands. That moral injury isn't some abstract concept—it's what happens when you have to choose who gets the last ECMO bed."

Rajiv looked up; eyes clouded. "We learned to build ICUs from scratch. Learned how to whisper hope through glass doors. And we learned that fear...doesn't go away. It just lives quietly beside you."

"And we learned," Eva added, "that silence is dangerous. That if we don't tell the story, others will rewrite it for us."

She reached into her bag and pulled out a slim notebook. The cover was plain, leather-bound.

"I've been writing about it," she said. "Not for publication. Just...to remember. For my kids. For me. For anyone who one day asks, What was it like?"

Rajiv stared at the notebook as though it were sacred.

"Tell them," He said quietly. "Tell them we weren't heroes as much as we were simply human. Tired, terrified, sometimes angry—and always trying."

"I will," she promised.

A nurse walked by, pushing a wheelchair. Behind them, a child laughed as cherry blossoms danced in the wind. Life, stubborn and persistent, continued.

"You think we're better prepared now?" Rajiv asked.

Eva shook her head. "Not really. The systems are still brittle. Staffing is worse. Public trust is frayed."

"But we know more," he said.

"We do. But knowledge isn't the same as change."

Rajiv stood up slowly, joints creaking. "Then maybe that's the work of the next five years."

They walked together toward the hospital, a little older, a little more worn, but still moving forward.

Behind them, the petals kept falling—quiet as memory, soft as grace.

About the Author

Arthur Lazarus, MD, MBA, is a healthcare consultant, certified physician executive, and nationally recognized author, speaker, and champion of physician leadership and wellness. He has broad experience in clinical practice and the health insurance industry, having led programs at Cigna and Humana. At Humana, Lazarus was vice president and corporate medical director of behavioral health operations in Louisville, Kentucky, and subsequently a population health medical director in the state of Florida.

Lazarus has also held leadership positions in several pharmaceutical companies, including Pfizer and AstraZeneca, conducting clinical trials and reviewing promotional material for medical accuracy and FDA compliance. He has published more than 450 articles and essays online and in scientific and professional journals and has written and edited over a dozen books, including many related to the field of narrative medicine.

Born in Philadelphia, Pennsylvania, Lazarus attended Boston University, where he graduated with a bachelor's degree in psychology with Distinction. He received his medical degree with Honors from Temple University School of Medicine, followed by a psychiatric residency at Temple University Hospital, where he was chief resident. After residency, Lazarus joined the faculty of Temple University School of Medicine, where he currently serves as adjunct professor of psychiatry. He also holds non-faculty appointments as Executive-in-Residence at Temple University Fox School of Business and Management, where he received his MBA degree, and Senior Fellow, Jefferson College of Population Health, Philadelphia, Pennsylvania.

Well known for his leadership and medical management skills, Lazarus is a sought-after presenter, mentor, teacher, and writer. He has shared his expertise and perspective at numerous local, national, and international meetings and seminars.

Lazarus is a past president of the American Association for Psychiatric Administration and Leadership, a former member of the board of directors of the American Association for Physician Leadership (AAPL), and a current member of the AAPL editorial review board. In 2010, the American Psychiatric Association honored Lazarus with the Administrative Psychiatry Award for his effectiveness as an administrator of major mental health programs and expanding the body of knowledge of management science in mental health services delivery systems.

Lazarus is among a select group of physicians in the United States who have been inducted into both the Alpha Omega Alpha medical honor society and the Beta Gamma Sigma honor society of collegiate schools of business.

Lazarus enjoys walking, biking, playing piano, and listening to music. He has been happily married to his wife, Cheryl, for over 40 years. They are the proud parents of four adult children and the grandparents of six young children.

Made in the USA
Monee, IL
03 November 2026

67384104R00213